KIDNEY DISEASE AND URINARY TRACT DISORDERS

SOURCEBOOK

FOURTH EDITION

Health Reference Series

KIDNEY DISEASE AND URINARY TRACT DISORDERS SOURCEBOOK

FOURTH EDITION

Basic Consumer Health Information about Kidney Health and Urinary Disorders, including the Causes, Symptoms, Diagnosis, and Treatment of Conditions Affecting the Kidneys, Ureters, Bladder, and Urethra

Along with Information on Managing Kidney Failure, Dialysis, Kidney Transplantation, Preventive Care, a Glossary of Related Terms, and a Directory of Resources for Additional Help and Support

OMNIGRAPHICS
An imprint of Infobase

* * *

OMNIGRAPHICS
An imprint of Infobase
8 The Green
Suite #19225
Dover, DE 19901
www.infobase.com
James Chambers, *Editorial Director*

* * *

ISBN 978-0-7808-2162-0
E-ISBN 978-0-7808-2163-7

Library of Congress Cataloging-in-Publication Data

Names: Chambers, James, editor.

Title: Kidney disease and urinary tract disorders sourcebook / edited by James Chambers.

Description: Fourth edition. | Dover, DE: Omnigraphics, an imprint of Infobase, [2025] | Series: Health reference series | Includes index. | Summary: "Provides health information about the kidneys and urinary system, with details on urinary tract infections, incontinence, congenital disorders, kidney stones, cancers of the kidneys and urinary tract, chronic kidney disease, kidney failure, dialysis, and kidney transplantation. Includes an index, a glossary, and a directory of resources for additional information"-- Provided by publisher.

Identifiers: LCCN 2024044911 (print) | LCCN 2024044912 (ebook) | ISBN 9780780821620 (acid-free paper) | ISBN 9780780821637 (eISBN)

Subjects: LCSH: Urinary organs--Popular works. | Urinary organs--Diseases--Popular works. | Kidneys--Diseases--Popular works. | Consumer education.

Classification: LCC RC900 .U745 2024 (print) | LCC RC900 (ebook) | DDC 616.6/1--dc23/eng/20241128

LC record available at https://lccn.loc.gov/2024044911

LC ebook record available at https://lccn.loc.gov/2024044912

Printed in the United States

Table of Contents

Part 3. Disorders of the Urinary Tract

Part 4. Disorders of the Bladder and Prostate

Part 5. Diagnostic Tests for Kidney Disease

Part 6. Kidney Failure: End-Stage Renal Disease

Part 7. Additional Help and Information

Preface

ABOUT THIS BOOK

Millions of Americans experience difficulties involving their kidneys, ureters, bladder, and urethra—the components of the urinary system. Problems can arise from illness, injury, genetic predisposition, or aging, resulting in conditions such as urinary incontinence, urinary tract infections, kidney stones, and kidney failure. According to 2023 data from the Centers for Disease Control and Prevention (CDC), more than one in seven U.S. adults—about 35.5 million people, or 14 percent—are estimated to have chronic kidney disease (CKD). Alarmingly, as many as 9 in 10 adults with CKD are unaware of their condition, and about one in three adults with severe CKD do not know they have it. While kidney disease and urinary tract disorders can significantly affect physical, emotional, and social well-being, advances in medical treatments offer promising solutions, helping those affected manage their conditions effectively. By understanding the risk factors associated with these disorders, individuals can make lifestyle adjustments and take preventive measures to preserve their urological health.

Kidney Disease and Urinary Tract Disorders Sourcebook, Fourth Edition provides comprehensive information about the urinary system and its components, including the kidneys, ureters, bladder, and urethra. It details the causes, symptoms, diagnosis, and treatment options for conditions such as chronic kidney disease, renal artery stenosis, urinary tract infections, kidney stones, and congenital genital and urinary disorders. Additionally, it discusses genetic and congenital kidney disorders, such as polycystic kidney disease, as well as cancers of the urinary system, including kidney and renal pelvis cancer. The book details diagnostic tests, including blood and urine tests, kidney biopsies, and imaging techniques used to detect kidney diseases. It explains treatment options such as dialysis and kidney transplantation, along with information on financial assistance available for kidney failure treatments. The book concludes with a glossary of related terms and a directory of resources offering information and support for individuals affected by kidney disease and urinary tract disorders.

HOW TO USE THIS BOOK

This book is divided into parts and chapters. Parts focus on broad areas of interest. Chapters are devoted to single topics within a part.

Part 1: Understanding the Urinary System provides a comprehensive overview of the urinary system, including the function and importance of the urinary tract. It explains kidney function and explores major risk factors for kidney disease, including diabetes, high blood pressure, obesity, and ethnic and racial factors.

Part 2: Disorders and Diseases of the Kidneys delves into chronic kidney disease, exploring its common causes, strategies for management, and prevention through healthy habits. It covers renal artery stenosis, childhood kidney diseases, and autoimmune-related disorders, such as lupus nephritis and Henoch-Schönlein purpura. The part also covers glomerular diseases, including nephrotic syndrome and IgA nephropathy, as well as genetic and congenital kidney disorders, such as polycystic kidney disease, Bartter syndrome, and Fabry disease.

Part 3: Disorders of the Urinary Tract examines urinary tract infections in different populations, including adults, children, and pregnant women. It also covers kidney stones, focusing on treatment, prevention, and dietary strategies to manage risk. Congenital urinary disorders in newborns, such as hypospadias and hydronephrosis, and urethral cancer are also discussed.

Part 4: Disorders of the Bladder and Prostate focuses on maintaining bladder health and addresses common issues such as urinary incontinence across demographics, including women, children, and older adults. It explores prostate problems, including prostatitis and benign prostatic hyperplasia, and discusses conditions such as urinary retention, interstitial cystitis, and cancers affecting the bladder and prostate.

Part 5: Diagnostic Tests for Kidney Disease outlines diagnostic tools for assessing kidney health, including blood tests such as creatinine and renal panel tests, urine tests, and imaging techniques. It explains how these tests are used to detect chronic kidney disease and other abnormalities, alongside procedures like kidney biopsies.

Part 6: Kidney Failure: End-Stage Renal Disease covers the management of kidney failure, including treatment options such as hemodialysis and peritoneal dialysis. It discusses kidney transplantation, conservative management strategies, and financial assistance for kidney failure treatments.

Part 7: Additional Help and Information includes a glossary of terms related to kidney disease and urinary tract disorders and a directory of resources for patients seeking support and further information.

BIBLIOGRAPHIC NOTE

This volume contains documents and excerpts from publications issued by the following U.S. government agencies: Centers for Disease Control and Prevention (CDC); Genetic and Rare Diseases Information Center (GARD); MedlinePlus; National Cancer Institute (NCI); National Institute of Diabetes and Digestive and Kidney Diseases (NIDDK); National Institute on Aging (NIA); National Institutes of Health (NIH); and Office on Women's Health (OWH).

ABOUT THE *HEALTH REFERENCE SERIES*

The *Health Reference Series* is designed to provide basic medical information for patients, families, caregivers, and the general public. Each volume provides comprehensive coverage on a particular topic. This is especially important for people who may be dealing with a newly diagnosed disease or a chronic disorder in themselves or in a family member. People looking for preventive guidance, information about disease warning signs, medical statistics, and risk factors for health problems will also find answers to their questions in the *Health Reference Series*. The *Series*, however, is not intended to serve as a tool for diagnosing illness, in prescribing treatments, or as a substitute for the physician-patient relationship. All people concerned about medical symptoms or the possibility of disease are encouraged to seek professional care from an appropriate health-care provider.

A NOTE ABOUT SPELLING AND STYLE

Health Reference Series editors use *Stedman's Medical Dictionary* as an authority for questions related to the spelling of medical terms and *The Chicago Manual of Style* for questions related to grammatical structures, punctuation, and other editorial concerns. Consistent adherence is not always possible, however, because the individual volumes within the *Series* include many documents from a wide variety of different producers, and the editor's primary goal is to present material from each source as accurately as is possible. This sometimes means that information in different chapters or sections may follow other guidelines and alternate spelling authorities. For example, occasionally a copyright holder may require that eponymous terms be shown in possessive forms (Crohn's disease vs. Crohn disease) or that British spelling norms be retained (leukaemia vs. leukemia).

HEALTH REFERENCE SERIES UPDATE POLICY

The inaugural book in the *Health Reference Series* was the first edition of *Cancer Sourcebook* published in 1989. Since then, the *Series* has been enthusiastically received by librarians and in the medical community. In order to maintain the standard of providing high-quality health information for the layperson, the editorial staff felt it was necessary to implement a policy of updating volumes when warranted.

Medical researchers have been making tremendous strides, and it is the purpose of the *Health Reference Series* to stay current with the most recent advances. Each decision to update a volume is made on an individual basis. Some of the considerations include how much new information is available and the feedback we receive from people who use the books. If there is a topic you would like to see added to the update list, or an area of medical concern you feel has not been adequately addressed, please write to: custserv@infobaselearning.com.

Part 1 | **Understanding the Urinary System**

Chapter 1 | The Function and Importance of the Urinary Tract

WHAT IS THE URINARY TRACT?

The urinary tract is the body's drainage system for removing urine, which is made up of wastes and extra fluid. For normal urination to occur, all body parts in the urinary tract need to work together in the correct order.

The urinary tract includes two kidneys, two ureters, a bladder, and a urethra (see Figure 1.1).

- **Kidneys**. Two bean-shaped organs, each about the size of a fist. They are located just below your rib cage, one on each side of your spine. Every day, your kidneys filter about 120–150 quarts of blood to remove wastes and balance fluids. This process produces about 1–2 quarts of urine per day.
- **Ureters**. The thin tubes of muscle that connect the kidneys to the bladder and carry urine to the bladder.
- **Bladder**. A hollow, muscular, balloon-shaped organ that expands as it fills with urine. The bladder sits in your pelvis between your hip bones. A normal bladder acts like a reservoir. It can hold 1.5–2 cups of urine. Although you do not control how your kidneys function, you can control when to empty your bladder. Bladder emptying is known as "urination."
- **Urethra**. A tube located at the bottom of the bladder that allows urine to exit the body during urination.

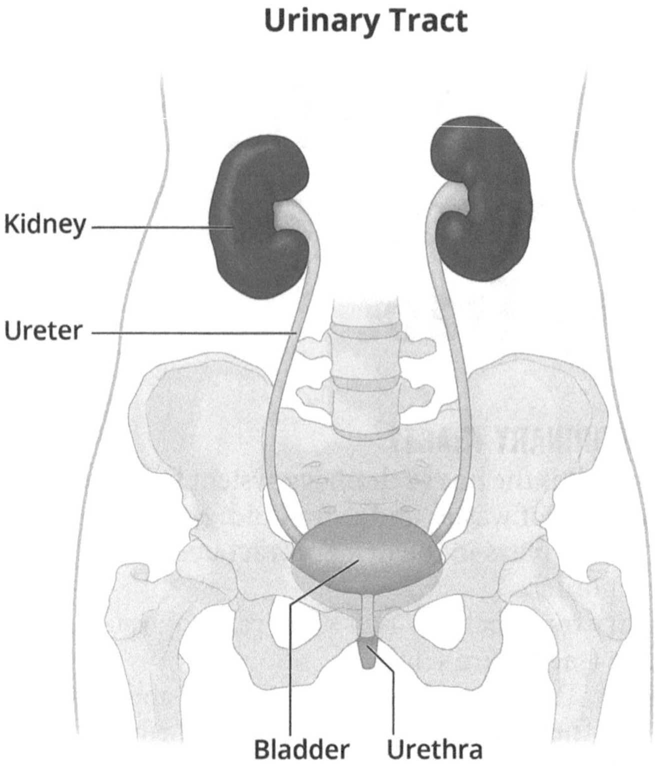

Figure 1.1. Urinary Tract

National Institute of Diabetes and Digestive and Kidney Diseases (NIDDK)

All parts of the urinary tract—the kidneys, ureters, bladder, and urethra—must work together to urinate normally. The urinary tract includes two sets of muscles that work together as a sphincter, closing off the urethra to keep urine in the bladder between trips to the bathroom.

The internal sphincter muscles of the bladder neck and urethra stay closed until your brain sends signals to urinate. The external sphincter muscles surround the internal sphincter and provide extra pressure to keep the urethra closed. You can consciously squeeze the external sphincter and the pelvic floor muscles to keep urine from leaking out.

HOW DOES URINATION OCCUR?

To urinate, your brain signals the sphincters to relax. Then it signals the muscular bladder wall to tighten, squeezing urine through the urethra and out of your bladder.

How often you need to urinate depends on how quickly your kidneys produce the urine that fills the bladder and how much urine your bladder can comfortably hold. The muscles of your bladder wall remain relaxed while the bladder fills with urine, and the sphincter muscles remain contracted to keep urine in the bladder. As your bladder fills up, signals sent to your brain tell you to find a toilet soon.

WHY IS THE URINARY TRACT IMPORTANT?

The urinary tract is important because it filters wastes and extra fluid from the bloodstream and removes them from the body.

WHAT AFFECTS THE AMOUNT OF URINE YOU PRODUCE?

The amount of urine you produce depends on many factors, such as the amount of liquid and food you consume and the amount of fluid you lose through sweating and breathing. Certain medicines, medical conditions, and types of food can also affect the amount of urine you produce. Children produce less urine than adults.

HOW CAN YOU KEEP YOUR URINARY TRACT HEALTHY?

You can help keep your urinary tract healthy by following some basic tips:

- **Drink enough liquids, especially water**. If you are healthy, try to drink six to eight 8-ounce glasses of liquid each day. You may need to drink more if you have kidney stones or bladder stones. At least half of your liquid intake should be water. You might need to drink less water if you have certain conditions, such as kidney failure or heart disease. Ask your health-care professional how much liquid is healthy for you.

- **Keep your bowels regular**. Regular bowel movements are important to your bladder health. You can promote both bowel health and bladder health by:
  - **Making healthy food choices**. You can keep your urinary tract healthy by sticking to an eating plan that includes lean proteins, whole grains, fiber-rich breads, nuts, colorful berries, fruits, and vegetables to promote regular bowel movements.
  - **Living a healthy lifestyle**. Get regular physical activity, limit your alcohol intake, cut down on caffeinated food and drinks, and do not smoke.
- **Go whenever you need to**. Often, people hold their urine because it is not a good time to go to the bathroom. However, holding in your urine for too long can weaken your bladder muscles and make it harder for your bladder to empty completely. Urine left in your bladder can allow bacteria to grow and make you more likely to develop a urinary tract infection (UTI).
- **Develop healthy bathroom habits**. Take enough time to fully empty your bladder when urinating—do not rush it. Urinate after sex to flush away bacteria that may have entered the urethra during sex. Clean the genital area before and after sex. If you are a woman, wipe from front to back, especially after a bowel movement, to keep bacteria from getting into the urethra.
- **Stay in tune with your body**. Pay attention to how often you feel the urge to urinate. Take note if you need to urinate more often than usual, if your urine leaks, if it becomes more difficult for you to begin urinating, or if you feel you are not able to completely empty your bladder. These changes may be early signs of different urinary tract problems. Talk with your health-care professional if you notice any of these signs. You may be able to prevent a condition from becoming more severe if you get help early on.
- **Do pelvic floor muscle exercises**. Pelvic floor exercises, also called "Kegel exercises," can keep your pelvic floor

muscles strong and maintain healthy bladder and bowel function. Both men and women can benefit from pelvic floor muscle exercises.

Maintaining a healthy urinary tract is essential for overall well-being. By following recommended practices and staying aware of bodily changes, individuals can support their urinary health and prevent complications.

CLINICAL TRIALS

The National Institute of Diabetes and Digestive and Kidney Diseases (NIDDK) conducts and supports clinical trials in many diseases and conditions, including urologic diseases. The trials look to find new ways to prevent, detect, or treat diseases and improve quality of life.[1]

[1] "The Urinary Tract and How It Works," National Institute of Diabetes and Digestive and Kidney Diseases (NIDDK), June 2020. Available online. URL: www.niddk.nih.gov/health-information/urologic-diseases/urinary-tract-how-it-works. Accessed October 14, 2024.

Chapter 2 | **Understanding Kidney Function**

WHAT ARE THE KIDNEYS?

The kidneys are two bean-shaped organs, each about the size of a fist. They are located just below the rib cage, one on each side of the spine.

Healthy kidneys filter about a half cup of blood every minute, removing wastes and extra water to make urine. The urine flows from the kidneys to the bladder through two thin tubes of muscle called "ureters," one on each side of the bladder. The bladder stores urine. The kidneys, ureters, and bladder are part of the urinary tract.

WHY ARE THE KIDNEYS IMPORTANT?

The kidneys remove wastes and extra fluid from the body. They also remove acid that is produced by the cells of the body and maintain a healthy balance of water, salts, and minerals—such as sodium, calcium, phosphorus, and potassium—in the blood.

Without this balance, nerves, muscles, and other tissues in the body may not work normally.

The kidneys also make hormones that help:

- control blood pressure
- make red blood cells
- keep bones strong and healthy

HOW DO THE KIDNEYS WORK?

Each kidney is made up of about a million filtering units called "nephrons." Each nephron includes a filter, called the "glomerulus," and a tubule. The nephrons work through a two-step process: the glomerulus filters the blood, and the tubule returns needed substances to the blood and removes wastes.

The Glomerulus Filters the Blood

As blood flows into each nephron, it enters a cluster of tiny blood vessels—the glomerulus. The glomerulus's thin walls allow smaller molecules, wastes, and fluid—mostly water—to pass into the tubule. Larger molecules, such as proteins and blood cells, stay in the blood vessel.

The Tubule Returns Needed Substances to the Blood and Removes Wastes

A blood vessel runs alongside the tubule. As the filtered fluid moves along the tubule, the blood vessel reabsorbs almost all the water, along with minerals and nutrients the body needs. The tubule helps remove excess acid from the blood. The remaining fluid and wastes in the tubule become urine.

HOW DOES BLOOD FLOW THROUGH THE KIDNEYS?

Blood flows into the kidney through the renal artery. This large blood vessel branches into smaller and smaller blood vessels until the blood reaches the nephrons. In the nephron, blood is filtered by the tiny blood vessels of the glomeruli and then flows out of the kidney through the renal vein (see Figure 2.1).

Blood circulates through the kidneys many times a day. In a single day, the kidneys filter about 150 quarts of blood. Most of the water and other substances that filter through the glomeruli are returned to the blood by the tubules. Only 1–2 quarts become urine. Children produce less urine than adults, and the amount produced depends on their age.[1]

---

[1] "Your Kidneys and How They Work," National Institute of Diabetes and Digestive and Kidney Diseases (NIDDK), June 2018. Available online. URL: www.niddk.nih.gov/health-information/kidney-disease/kidneys-how-they-work. Accessed October 15, 2024.

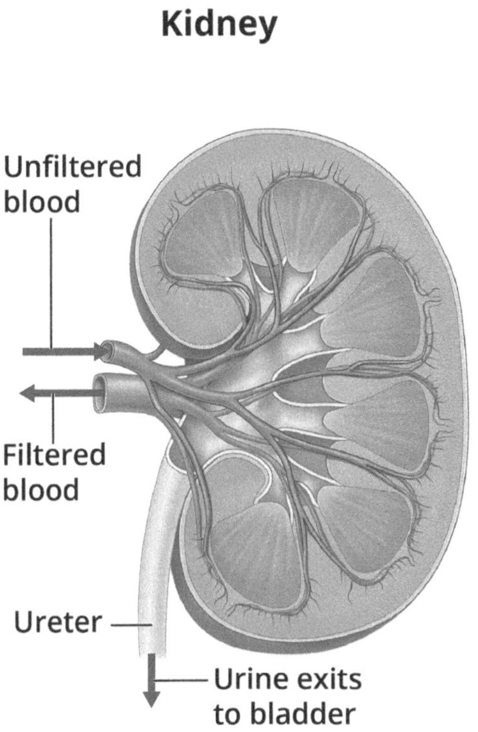

Figure 2.1. Kidney

National Institute of Diabetes and Digestive and Kidney Diseases (NIDDK)

Chapter 3 | Major Risk Factors for Kidney Disease

Chapter Contents

Section 3.1 | Diabetes and Kidney Disease

WHAT IS CHRONIC KIDNEY DISEASE?

Chronic kidney disease (CKD) often develops slowly and with few symptoms. Many people do not realize they have CKD until it is advanced. At that point, they need dialysis (a treatment that filters the blood) or a kidney transplant to survive.

If you have diabetes, get your kidneys checked regularly. Your doctor will do this with simple blood and urine tests. Regular testing is your best chance to identify CKD early if it develops. Early treatment is most effective and can help prevent additional health problems.

CKD is common in people with diabetes. Approximately one in three adults with diabetes have CKD. Both type 1 and type 2 diabetes can cause kidney disease.

HOW DIABETES CAUSES CHRONIC KIDNEY DISEASE

Each kidney is made up of millions of tiny filters called "nephrons." Over time, high blood sugar from diabetes can damage blood vessels in the kidneys and nephrons. Many people with diabetes also develop high blood pressure (HBP), which can damage the kidneys.

CKD takes a long time to develop and usually does not have any signs or symptoms in the early stages. One will not know they have CKD unless their doctor checks for it.

TIPS FOR HEALTHY KIDNEYS

You can help keep your kidneys healthy by managing blood sugar, blood pressure, and cholesterol levels. This is also very important for heart and blood vessel health. High blood sugar, blood pressure, and cholesterol levels are all risk factors for heart disease and stroke.

- Keep blood sugar levels in the target range as much as possible.
- Get an A1C test at least twice a year. Ask your doctor how often is right for you.

- Keep blood pressure below 140/90 mm Hg (or the target set by your doctor).
- Stay in the target cholesterol range.
- Eat foods lower in sodium.
- Eat more fruits and vegetables.
- Be physically active.
- Take medicines as directed.

PREDIABETES AND CHRONIC KIDNEY DISEASE

With prediabetes, blood sugar levels are higher than normal but not high enough for a type 2 diabetes diagnosis. Prediabetes is a serious health condition that increases the risk of developing type 2 diabetes, heart disease, and stroke. If one has prediabetes, taking action to prevent type 2 diabetes is an important step in preventing CKD.

- Losing a small amount of weight if overweight.
- Getting regular physical activity.[1]

Section 3.2 | **High Blood Pressure and Kidney Disease**

WHAT IS HIGH BLOOD PRESSURE?

Blood pressure is the force of blood pushing against blood vessel walls as the heart pumps out blood. High blood pressure (HBP), also called "hypertension," is an increase in the amount of force that blood places on blood vessels as it moves through the body.

HOW DOES HIGH BLOOD PRESSURE AFFECT THE KIDNEYS?

High blood pressure can constrict and narrow the blood vessels, eventually damaging and weakening them throughout the body, including the kidneys. The narrowing reduces blood flow.

---

[1] "Chronic Kidney Disease," Centers for Disease Control and Prevention (CDC), May 15, 2024. Available online. URL: www.cdc.gov/diabetes/diabetes-complications/diabetes-and-chronic-kidney-disease.html. Accessed October 15, 2024.

If the kidneys' blood vessels are damaged, they may no longer work properly. When this happens, the kidneys are not able to remove all wastes and extra fluid from the body. Extra fluid in the blood vessels can raise blood pressure even more, creating a dangerous cycle and causing more damage, leading to kidney failure.

HOW COMMON ARE HIGH BLOOD PRESSURE AND KIDNEY DISEASE?

High blood pressure is the second leading cause of kidney failure in the United States after diabetes (see Figure 3.1). Almost one in two U.S. adults—or about 108 million people—have HBP. More than one in seven U.S. adults—or about 37 million people—may have chronic kidney disease (CKD).

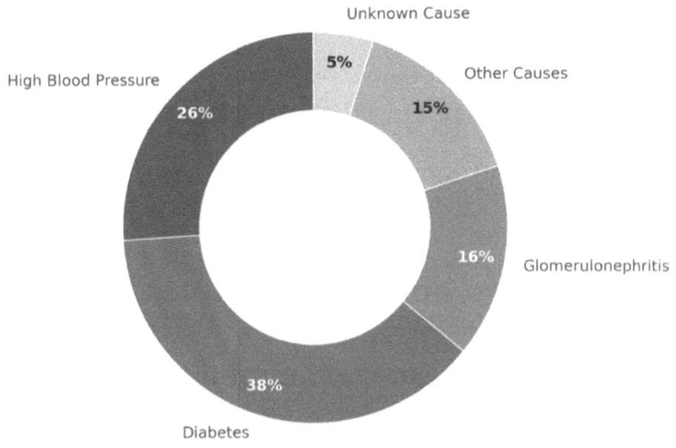

Figure 3.1. Causes of Kidney Disease

National Institute of Diabetes and Digestive and Kidney Diseases (NIDDK)

WHO IS MORE LIKELY TO HAVE HIGH BLOOD PRESSURE OR KIDNEY DISEASE?

High Blood Pressure

- **Age.** Blood pressure tends to increase with age as blood vessels naturally thicken and stiffen over time.

- **Family history**. HBP tends to run in families.
- **Unhealthy lifestyle**. Unhealthy habits such as consuming too much sodium (salt), drinking excessive alcoholic beverages, or not being physically active can increase the risk of HBP.
- **Ethnicity**. More common in African-American adults than in Caucasian, Hispanic, or Asian adults.
- **Gender**. Men are more likely to develop HBP before age 55; women are more likely to develop it after age 55.

Kidney Disease

- **Being diabetic.**
- **Family history**. A family history of kidney failure.
- **Race or ethnicity**. African Americans, Hispanics, and American Indians tend to have a greater risk for CKD.

HBP can be both a cause and a result of kidney disease.

WHAT ARE THE SYMPTOMS OF HIGH BLOOD PRESSURE AND KIDNEY DISEASE?

Most people with HBP do not have symptoms. In rare cases, it can cause headaches.

Early CKD may also not have symptoms. As kidney disease worsens, some people may experience swelling, called "edema." Edema occurs when the kidneys cannot eliminate extra fluid and salt, which can manifest in the legs, feet, ankles, or, less frequently, in the hands or face.

Symptoms of advanced kidney disease can include:

- loss of appetite, nausea, or vomiting
- drowsiness, feeling tired, or sleep problems
- headaches or trouble concentrating
- increased or decreased urination
- generalized itching or numbness, dry skin, or darkened skin
- weight loss
- muscle cramps
- chest pain or shortness of breath

HOW DO HEALTH-CARE PROFESSIONALS DIAGNOSE HIGH BLOOD PRESSURE AND KIDNEY DISEASE?

High Blood Pressure

Blood pressure test results are expressed as two numbers separated by a slash. The top number is called "systolic pressure" and represents the pressure as the heart beats and pushes blood through the blood vessels. The bottom number is called "diastolic pressure" and represents the pressure as blood vessels relax between heartbeats.

Health-care professionals diagnose HBP if blood pressure readings are consistently higher than 130/80 when tested repeatedly in a health-care office. Blood pressure is measured with a blood pressure cuff, which can also be used at home.

Kidney Disease

To check for kidney disease, health-care professionals use:

- a blood test that checks how well the kidneys filter the blood, called "GFR," which stands for "glomerular filtration rate"
- a urine test to check for albumin, a protein that can pass into the urine when the kidneys are damaged

If kidney disease is present, health-care professionals will use the same two tests to monitor the condition.

HOW CAN ONE PREVENT OR SLOW THE PROGRESSION OF KIDNEY DISEASE FROM HIGH BLOOD PRESSURE?

The best way to slow or prevent kidney disease from HBP is to take steps to lower blood pressure. These steps include a combination of medicines and lifestyle changes, such as:

- being physically active
- maintaining a healthy weight
- quitting smoking
- managing stress
- following a healthy diet, including less sodium (salt) intake

High blood pressure can worsen kidney conditions. Discuss individual blood pressure goals and the frequency of blood pressure checks with a health-care professional.

HOW DOES EATING, DIET, AND NUTRITION AFFECT HIGH BLOOD PRESSURE AND KIDNEY DISEASE?

Following a healthy eating plan can help lower blood pressure. Reducing sodium intake is a crucial part of any healthy eating plan. Health-care professionals may recommend the "Dietary Approaches to Stop Hypertension" (DASH) eating plan, which focuses on fruits, vegetables, whole grains, and other heart-healthy foods that are lower in sodium. The DASH eating plan is characterized by several key features:

- It is low in fat and cholesterol.
- It includes fat-free or low-fat milk and dairy products, fish, poultry, and nuts.
- It recommends consuming less red meat, sweets, added sugars, and sugar-containing beverages.
- It is rich in nutrients, protein, and fiber.

A registered dietitian can assist in tailoring a diet to address kidney disease. For those with congestive heart failure or edema, a diet low in sodium can help reduce edema and lower blood pressure. Reducing saturated fat and cholesterol can help control elevated lipid levels in the blood.

People with advanced kidney disease should consult a health-care professional regarding their diet.

WHAT SHOULD ONE AVOID EATING IF HIGH BLOOD PRESSURE OR KIDNEY DISEASE IS PRESENT?

If kidney disease is present, avoid foods and beverages that are high in sodium. Additional steps to meet blood pressure goals may include eating heart-healthy and low-sodium meals, quitting smoking, being active, getting adequate sleep, and taking prescribed medications. Limit alcoholic drinks—no more than two per day for men and one per day for women—as excessive consumption can raise blood pressure.

A health-care professional may recommend moderate or reduced protein intake. Proteins break down into waste products that the kidneys filter from the blood. Consuming excess protein may burden the kidneys and accelerate functional decline. However, insufficient protein intake can lead to malnutrition.

For individuals on a restricted protein diet due to kidney disease, a health-care professional will monitor nutrient levels through blood tests.[1]

Section 3.3 | **Obesity and Kidney Disease**

OBESITY

Obesity is a chronic disease affecting more than one in three adults and about 17 percent of children and adolescents in the United States. More than one in three adults is overweight. Being overweight or obese increases the risk of type 2 diabetes, heart disease, kidney disease, stroke, fatty liver disease, and other health issues.

A healthy eating plan and regular physical activity can help people lose weight and maintain it over the long term.

BODY MASS INDEX

Body mass index (BMI) estimates whether an individual has a healthy weight, is overweight, or obese. Adults can use a BMI calculator (www.nhlbi.nih.gov/health/educational/lose_wt/BMI/bmicalc.htm) to estimate their BMI.

BMI is calculated based on height and weight. It does not directly measure body fat. Therefore, it may not accurately assess health risks related to excess body fat. For example:

- **Individuals who are very muscular, such as bodybuilders, may have a high BMI without a significant amount of body fat.**

[1] "High Blood Pressure and Kidney Disease," National Institute of Diabetes and Digestive and Kidney Diseases (NIDDK), March 2020. Available online. URL: www.niddk.nih.gov/health-information/kidney-disease/high-blood-pressure. Accessed October 15, 2024.

- **Some people of Asian descent tend to store extra body fat around their waist.** Storing extra fat around the abdomen can increase their risk for weight-related health problems, even if their BMI is not high.
- **Older adults tend to lose bone and muscle and gain body fat as they age.** Gaining extra body fat can increase the risk of health problems, even if the BMI does not change.

KIDNEY DISEASE

Kidney disease means the kidneys are damaged and cannot filter blood as they should. Obesity raises the risk of developing diabetes and high blood pressure, the most common causes of chronic kidney disease (CKD). Even without diabetes or high blood pressure, obesity may increase the risk of developing CKD and accelerate its progression.

Losing weight may help in preventing or delaying CKD. In the early stages of CKD, consuming healthy foods and beverages, being active, and losing excess weight may slow the disease's progress and keep the kidneys healthier longer.

MAINTAINING WEIGHT LOSS

Keeping weight off can be challenging. Metabolism slows down during weight loss, and fewer calories are needed at a new, lower weight. Changes in hormones and other factors may also make it hard to maintain weight loss.

Stick to a Healthy Eating Plan

It is crucial to continue making healthy food choices and following an eating plan as a lifelong habit. Finding healthy food options that are preferred and enjoyable will make adherence to an eating plan more likely.

Continue Regular Physical Activity

Engaging in regular physical activity may help keep weight off. To prevent weight regain, at least 300 minutes a week of moderate-intensity physical activity is recommended. Making regular physical activity a lifelong habit is essential.

Keep Track of Weight

Regularly weighing and keeping a record of changes in weight may help one stay focused and address setbacks in meeting goals. Experiencing setbacks does not equate to failure. The key is to resume the plan as soon as possible.[1]

HOW WEIGHT MANAGEMENT MEDICATIONS WORK

Prescription medications for treating overweight and obesity work in various ways. For example, some medications may help in feeling less hungry or full sooner. Others may make it harder for the body to absorb fat from the foods eaten.

WHO MIGHT BENEFIT FROM WEIGHT MANAGEMENT MEDICATIONS?

Weight management medications are intended to help those with health problems related to overweight or obesity. Health-care professionals use BMI to determine whether medication might be beneficial. Medication may be prescribed to treat overweight or obesity if an adult has a BMI of:

- 30 or greater
- 27 or greater, with weight-related health problems such as high blood pressure or type 2 diabetes

Weight management medications are not suitable for everyone with a high BMI. Losing weight with a lifestyle program that changes behaviors and improves eating and physical activity habits may be possible. A lifestyle program may also address other factors that contribute to weight gain, such as eating triggers and insufficient sleep.

[1] "Health Risks of Overweight and Obesity," National Institute of Diabetes and Digestive and Kidney Diseases (NIDDK), May 2023. Available online. URL: www.niddk.nih.gov/health-information/weight-management/adult-overweight-obesity/health-risks. Accessed October 18, 2024.

CAN CHILDREN OR TEENAGERS TAKE WEIGHT MANAGEMENT MEDICATIONS?

The U.S. Food and Drug Administration (FDA) has approved four weight management medications for individuals aged 12 and older:

- orlistat (Xenical)
- liraglutide (Saxenda)
- phentermine-topiramate (Qsymia)
- semaglutide (Wegovy)

A fifth prescription medication, setmelanotide (IMCIVREE), is approved for children aged six years and older who have rare genetic disorders causing obesity.[2]

Section 3.4 | **Ethnic and Racial Factors in Kidney Disease**

Chronic kidney disease (CKD) affects more than one in seven U.S. adults—an estimated 37 million Americans. For Americans with diabetes or high blood pressure (HBP)—the two most common causes of kidney disease—the risk for CKD is even greater. Nearly one in three people with diabetes and one in five people with HBP have kidney disease. Other risk factors for developing kidney disease include heart disease and a family history of kidney failure.

Despite the prevalence of kidney disease in the United States, as many as nine in ten adults who have CKD are not aware they have the disease. Early-stage kidney disease usually has no symptoms, and many people do not realize they have CKD until it is very advanced. Kidney disease often worsens over time and may lead to kidney failure and other health problems, such as stroke or heart attack. Approximately 2 in 1,000 Americans are living with end-stage kidney disease (ESKD)—kidney failure that is treated with a kidney transplant or dialysis.

[2] "Prescription Medications to Treat Overweight and Obesity," National Institute of Diabetes and Digestive and Kidney Diseases (NIDDK), June 2024. Available online. URL: www.niddk.nih.gov/health-information/weight-management/prescription-medications-treat-overweight-obesity. Accessed October 18, 2024.

KEY KIDNEY DISEASE STATISTICS

Chronic Kidney Disease

According to the Centers for Disease Control and Prevention's (CDC) Chronic Kidney Disease in the United States, 2021 report:

- CKD is slightly more common in women (14%) than in men (12%).
- About 16 percent of non-Hispanic Black adults have CKD.
- Approximately 13 percent of non-Hispanic white adults have CKD.
- About 13 percent of non-Hispanic Asian adults have CKD.
- Approximately 14 percent of Hispanic adults have CKD.
- CKD is most common among people aged 65 or older (38%), followed by those aged 45–64 (12%), and those aged 18–44 (6%).

End-Stage Kidney Disease

According to the United States Renal Data System 2020 Annual Data Report:

- Nearly 808,000 people in the United States are living with ESKD, also known as "end-stage renal disease" (ESRD), with 69 percent on dialysis and 31 percent with a kidney transplant.
- Men are 1.6 times more likely to develop ESKD than women.
- Compared with white people:
    - Black people are nearly four times more likely to develop ESKD.
    - Hispanic people and Native American people are more than twice as likely to develop ESKD.
    - Asian people are 1.4 times more likely to develop ESKD.
- Black people make up about 13 percent of the total population but account for 30 percent of the people with ESKD in the United States.

- Black people are more likely to have ESKD caused by high blood pressure, also called "hypertension," than white or Hispanic people.
- Since 2000, the number of Hispanic, Native Hawaiian and Other Pacific Islander, and Asian people with kidney failure has more than tripled in each racial/ethnic group.
- Hispanic people are more likely to have ESKD caused by diabetes than white or Black people.
- White people were more likely to receive a transplant by five years (63.2%) than Black, Hispanic, and Asian people (approximately 50%) and Native American and Native Hawaiian/Pacific Islander people (approximately 40%).

MORTALITY

According to the United States Renal Data System 2022 Annual Data Report:

- In 2020, the adjusted mortality rate was more than twice as high among Medicare beneficiaries aged 66 years or older with CKD (103.9 per 1,000 person-years) than among those without CKD (47.9 per 1,000).
- Adjusted mortality among people with CKD increased from 91.7 per 1,000 in 2019 to 100.6 per 1,000 in 2020, with a greater increase among Black and Hispanic people with CKD than among their white counterparts.
- Mortality increased by 23 percent among Black people.
- Mortality increased by approximately 12 percent among Hispanic people.
- Mortality increased by approximately 9 percent among white people.[1]

[1] "Kidney Disease Statistics for the United States," National Institute of Diabetes and Digestive and Kidney Diseases (NIDDK), May 2023. Available online. URL: www.niddk.nih.gov/health-information/kidney-disease/race-ethnicity. Accessed October 14, 2024.

Chapter 4 | Chronic Kidney Disease in the United States

When people develop chronic kidney disease (CKD), their kidneys become damaged and may not clean the blood as well as healthy kidneys over time. If kidneys do not function well, toxic waste and excess fluid can accumulate in the body, potentially leading to high blood pressure (HBP), heart disease, stroke, and early death. However, people with CKD and those at risk for CKD can take steps to protect their kidneys with the help of their health-care providers.

More than one in seven U.S. adults—about 35.5 million people, or 14 percent—are estimated to have CKD. As many as 9 in 10 adults with CKD do not know they have it. About one in three adults with severe CKD do not know they have CKD.

CHRONIC KIDNEY DISEASE BY AGE, SEX, AND RACE/ETHNICITY

According to current estimates:

- CKD is more common in people aged 65 years or older (34%) than in people aged 45–64 years (12%) or 18–44 years (6%).
- CKD is slightly more common in women (14%) than in men (12%).
- CKD is more common in non-Hispanic Black adults (20%) than in non-Hispanic Asian adults (14%) or non-Hispanic white adults (12%).
- About 14 percent of Hispanic adults have CKD.

CHRONIC KIDNEY DISEASE RISK FACTORS

Diabetes and HBP are the more common causes of CKD in most adults. Other risk factors include heart disease, obesity, a family history of CKD, inherited kidney disorders, past damage to the kidneys, and older age.

WAYS TO PREVENT CHRONIC KIDNEY DISEASE

Manage risk factors for CKD:

- high blood sugar levels
- high blood pressure

Keeping a healthy body weight through a balanced diet and physical activity can help manage blood pressure and blood sugar levels in people with diabetes or in those at risk of developing type 2 diabetes.

Treatment to Lower Blood Sugar

Newer blood sugar–lowering medicines, such as GLP1 receptor agonists, SGLT2 inhibitors, and DPP-4 inhibitors, have been approved by the U.S. Food and Drug Administration (FDA). These medicines are recommended for people with both diabetes and CKD to reduce risks for kidney disease progression or cardiovascular complications. Percentages of adults with both CKD and diagnosed diabetes who are prescribed these blood sugar-lowering medicines differ by age and race/ethnicity:

- Adults with both CKD and diagnosed diabetes are more likely to be prescribed newer blood sugar-lowering medicines if they are aged 45–64 years (21%) and 65 years or older (18%) than if they are aged 18–44 years (11%).
- Adult women with both CKD and diagnosed diabetes are about as likely to be prescribed newer blood sugar-lowering medicines (18%) as adult men (15%).
- Non-Hispanic white adults (20%) and non-Hispanic Black adults (20%) with both CKD and diagnosed diabetes are more likely to be prescribed newer blood sugar-lowering medicines than Hispanic adults (8%) or non-Hispanic Asian adults (6%).

Treatment to Lower Blood Pressure

Blood pressure-lowering medicines are recommended for people with both diabetes and CKD. Percentages of adults with both CKD and diagnosed diabetes who are prescribed blood pressure-lowering medicines differ by age, sex, and race/ethnicity:

- Adults with both CKD and diagnosed diabetes are more likely to be prescribed blood pressure medicines if they are aged 45–64 years (63%) or 65 years or older (71%) than if they are aged 18–44 years (30%).
- Adult women with both CKD and diagnosed diabetes are more likely to be prescribed blood pressure medicines (53%) than adult men (45%).
- Non-Hispanic Black adults with both CKD and diagnosed diabetes are more likely to be prescribed blood pressure medicines (61%) than non-Hispanic white adults (45%) or non-Hispanic Asian adults (36%).
- About 45 percent of Hispanic adults with both CKD and diagnosed diabetes are prescribed blood pressure medicines.

TESTING AND TREATMENT

Test for CKD regularly in people who have diabetes, HBP, or other risk factors for CKD. People with CKD may not feel ill or notice any symptoms until CKD is advanced. The only way to determine if someone has CKD is through simple blood and urine tests. The blood test checks for the level of creatinine, a waste product produced by muscles, to see how well the kidneys work. The urine test checks for protein, which may indicate kidney damage.

Following a healthy diet and taking medicine for diabetes, medicine for HBP, and other medicines to protect the kidneys may help prevent CKD from worsening and may prevent other health problems such as heart disease.

CHRONIC KIDNEY DISEASE-RELATED HEALTH PROBLEMS

As CKD worsens over time, related health problems become more likely. However, CKD-related health problems can improve with treatment.

Heart Disease and Stroke

Having CKD increases the chances of having heart disease and stroke. Managing HBP, blood sugar, and cholesterol levels—all factors that increase the risk for heart disease and stroke—is very important for people with CKD.

Early Death

Adults with CKD are at a higher risk of dying earlier than adults of similar age without CKD.

Health Problems due to Low Kidney Function

- anemia or low red blood cell count, which can cause fatigue and weakness
- extra fluid in the body, which can cause HBP, swelling in the legs, or shortness of breath
- a weakened immune system, which makes it easier to develop infections
- loss of appetite or nausea
- decreased sexual response
- confusion, problems with memory and thinking, or depression
- low calcium levels and high phosphorus levels in the blood, which can cause bone disease and heart disease
- high potassium levels in the blood, which can cause an irregular or abnormal heartbeat and lead to death

Kidney Failure

Kidney failure occurs when kidney damage is severe and kidney function is very low. Dialysis or a kidney transplant is then needed for survival. Kidney failure treated with dialysis or a kidney transplant is referred to as "end-stage kidney disease" (ESKD). CKD is more likely to lead to kidney failure, especially in older adults, if the kidneys are damaged due to unmanaged risk factors, repeated kidney infections, or drugs or toxins that are harmful to the kidneys. Social factors, such as lower income and related factors of food insecurity and poorer access to quality health care, are also associated with worsening CKD. However, not everyone with CKD develops kidney failure. If CKD is detected early, treatment may slow the decline in kidney function and delay kidney failure. In some cases, though, kidney failure develops even with treatment.

PEOPLE WITH CHRONIC KIDNEY DISEASE CAN LOWER THEIR RISK FOR KIDNEY FAILURE

Learning about CKD from a primary care doctor or a kidney doctor (nephrologist) can enhance understanding of treatment options and kidney protection. People with glomerulonephritis, polycystic kidney disease, or other kidney diseases should discuss specific treatment options with a kidney doctor.

To maintain kidney health and manage CKD, it is essential to follow these key steps:

- Monitor and manage blood sugar and blood pressure.
    - Have blood sugar and blood pressure checked regularly.
    - Use medicines if prescribed to lower blood sugar and blood pressure.
- Make lifestyle changes (e.g., healthy eating, physical activity) to prevent further kidney damage.
- Meet with a dietitian to create a kidney-healthy eating plan that is low in salt and fat and has the appropriate amount and sources of protein. As CKD progresses, the plan may also include limiting phosphorus and potassium.
- Use medicines as directed to slow the decline in kidney function.
- Stop smoking or do not start smoking.
- Avoid exposures that can harm the kidneys or cause kidney function to suddenly deteriorate:
    - over-the-counter pain medicines such as ibuprofen and naproxen, which are also called "nonsteroidal anti-inflammatory drugs"
    - some antibiotics
    - certain herbal supplements
    - excessive alcohol intake[1]

[1] "Chronic Kidney Disease in the United States, 2023," Centers for Disease Control and Prevention (CDC), 2023. Available online. URL: www.cdc.gov/kidney-disease/media/pdfs/CKD-Factsheet-H.pdf. Accessed October 14, 2024.

Chapter 5 | **Electrolyte Balance and Adequate Hydration for Kidney Health**

WHAT ARE ELECTROLYTES?

Electrolytes are minerals that carry an electric charge when dissolved in water or body fluids, including blood. The electric charge can be positive or negative. You have electrolytes in your blood, urine, tissues, and other body fluids.

Electrolytes are important because they help:

- balance the amount of water in your body
- maintain your body's acid/base (pH) level
- move nutrients into your cells
- remove wastes from your cells
- support your muscle and nerve function
- keep your heart rate and rhythm steady
- maintain stable blood pressure
- ensure your bones and teeth remain healthy

TYPES OF ELECTROLYTES IN THE BODY

The main electrolytes in your body include:

- **Bicarbonate.** Helps maintain the body's acid and base balance (pH) and plays a role in moving carbon dioxide through the bloodstream.

- **Calcium**. Essential for making and keeping bones and teeth strong.
- **Chloride**. Helps control the amount of fluid in the body, maintain healthy blood volume, and regulate blood pressure.
- **Magnesium**. Supports proper muscle, nerve, and heart function, as well as controls blood pressure and blood glucose (blood sugar) levels.
- **Phosphate**. Works with calcium to build strong bones and teeth.
- **Potassium**. Essential for the proper functioning of cells, heart, and muscles.
- **Sodium**. Regulates fluid levels in the body and supports nerve and muscle function.

You obtain these electrolytes from the foods you eat and the fluids you drink.

WHAT IS AN ELECTROLYTE IMBALANCE?

An electrolyte imbalance occurs when the level of one or more electrolytes in your body is too low or too high. This imbalance can occur when the amount of water in your body changes. The amount of water you take in should equal the amount you lose. If something disrupts this balance, you may experience either too little water (dehydration) or too much water (overhydration). Some common reasons for an electrolyte imbalance include:

- certain medications
- severe vomiting and/or diarrhea
- heavy sweating
- heart, liver, or kidney problems
- not drinking enough fluids, especially during intense exercise or in very hot weather
- drinking excessive amounts of water

Table 5.1 provides an overview of common types of electrolyte imbalances, detailing conditions that occur when electrolyte levels are either too low or too high.

Table 5.1. Types of Electrolyte Imbalances

Electrolyte	**Too Low**	**Too High**
Bicarbonate	Acidosis	Alkalosis
Calcium	Hypocalcemia	Hypercalcemia
Chloride	Hypochloremia	Hyperchloremia
Magnesium	Hypomagnesemia	Hypermagnesemia
Phosphate	Hypophosphatemia	Hyperphosphatemia
Potassium	Hypokalemia	Hyperkalemia
Sodium	Hyponatremia	Hypernatremia

DIAGNOSIS OF ELECTROLYTE IMBALANCES

An electrolyte panel test can check the levels of your body's main electrolytes. A related test, the anion gap blood test, assesses whether your electrolytes are out of balance or if your blood is too acidic or not acidic enough.

TREATMENTS FOR ELECTROLYTE IMBALANCES

The treatment for an electrolyte imbalance depends on which electrolytes are out of balance, whether there is too little or too much, and the underlying cause of the imbalance. In minor cases, you may only need to adjust your diet. In other cases, more specific treatments may be required. For example:

- **If you have insufficient levels of electrolytes, you may receive electrolyte replacement therapy**. This involves administering more of that electrolyte, either through a supplement you swallow or drink, or it may be given intravenously (by IV).
- **If you have excessive levels of an electrolyte, your provider may give you medications or fluids (either by mouth or IV) to help eliminate that electrolyte from your body**. In severe cases, you may require dialysis to filter out the electrolyte.[1]

[1] MedlinePlus, "Fluid and Electrolyte Balance," National Institutes of Health (NIH), May 15, 2024. Available online. URL: https://medlineplus.gov/fluidandelectrolytebalance.html. Accessed October 16, 2024.

IMPORTANCE OF HYDRATION

About two-thirds of your body weight consists of water. All your cells need water to function properly. Water is also the base for various body fluids, including saliva, blood, urine, sweat, and joint fluid. No living organism can survive without water.

How can you tell if you are drinking enough? Your body loses water through sweating, urination, and even when you breathe out. Therefore, you need to consume enough water to replace what you lose. Insufficient water intake can lead to dehydration.

SIGNS OF DEHYDRATION

Signs that you may be becoming dehydrated include:

- intense thirst
- headaches
- dry mouth or skin
- darker urine, indicating your body is trying to conserve water

Drinking fluids should be sufficient to alleviate mild dehydration.

If dehydration becomes severe, it can lead to confusion, fainting, an inability to urinate, and rapid heartbeat and breathing. At this stage, it can be life-threatening, and you should seek medical attention immediately. Drinking liquids may not be adequate to replenish your body's fluids. You may need intravenous fluids through a needle or tube inserted into a vein.

LONG-TERM HEALTH IMPLICATIONS OF DEHYDRATION

Recent research funded by the National Institutes of Health (NIH) suggests that avoiding dehydration may not be the only reason to ensure adequate fluid intake. Dr. Natalia Dmitrieva, a heart researcher at NIH, has studied the long-term effects of insufficient hydration. In one study, her team discovered that middle-aged people who were not adequately hydrated were at a higher risk of developing chronic diseases, including heart failure, diabetes, chronic lung disease, and dementia. These people were also more likely to age faster and have a shorter lifespan. Therefore, staying well hydrated may help you maintain better health as you age.

RECOMMENDATIONS FOR FLUID INTAKE

The best way to avoid dehydration is to ensure you drink enough fluids every day. Ideally, your fluid intake should come from water or other low-calorie beverages, such as plain coffee, tea, or sparkling/flavored waters. Nutritional beverages, such as milk or milk alternatives and 100 percent vegetable juice, are also good options. Relying on soda, sports drinks, or other sugary beverages for most of your fluids can add unnecessary calories to your diet and provide little nutritional value.

The amount of fluid you should drink each day depends on various factors, including your age, where you live, and your body weight. Your body does not always lose water at the same rate; for example, when you exercise or are active in hot weather, you sweat more and need to drink more. However, experts generally recommend that women drink around 9 cups of fluids daily and men drink around 13 cups on average.

Certain conditions, such as diabetes or chronic kidney disease, and some medications can increase urination. You also lose significant amounts of water when you vomit, have diarrhea, or have a fever. In these cases, you need to drink more water to prevent dehydration.[2]

[2] *NIH News in Health*, "Hydrating for Health," National Institutes of Health (NIH), May 2023. Available online. URL: https://newsinhealth.nih.gov/2023/05/hydrating-health. Accessed October 16, 2024.

Chapter 6 | Nutrition for Children with Chronic Kidney Disease

WHY IS NUTRITION IMPORTANT FOR CHILDREN WITH CHRONIC KIDNEY DISEASE?

Eating the right foods in the right amounts may improve a child's growth, help them feel better, and prevent or delay health problems from chronic kidney disease (CKD).

Healthy kidneys balance the salts and minerals—such as calcium, phosphorus, sodium, and potassium—in the blood. When a child has kidney disease, their kidneys are damaged and cannot filter blood as they should. What a child eats and drinks can help maintain a healthy balance of salts and minerals in their body.

Eating right can also enhance the effectiveness of a child's CKD medicines.

A child's health-care team will work with parents to create an eating plan with the right foods and nutrients in the right amounts for proper growth. The team may suggest changes in both the amount and types of food a child needs as they get older or if their kidney disease worsens. Learning about nutrients in food will help parents understand what changes need to be made to a child's diet. It is essential to consult with the health-care team before making any significant changes to a child's diet.

WHY ARE CALORIES IMPORTANT?

Food provides the energy a child needs to grow and be active. Children with CKD tend to avoid eating because they do not feel hungry. Parents should talk with their child's kidney specialist or dietitian to ensure the child is getting enough calories for proper growth and to fight infections.

Children's calorie needs change depending on their age, height, and weight. A child's health-care team will determine their daily calorie needs, which will change as they grow.

To ensure proper growth, a health-care professional will compare a child's height and weight against growth charts that show the normal ranges of growth for children by age. If a child is not growing well, the health-care team can suggest healthy ways to add calories to their diet. Feeding tubes—thin, flexible tubes that carry liquid food into the stomach or small intestine—are often used for infants and, occasionally, situations arise in which older children and teenagers may also benefit from them.

WHY IS KNOWING ABOUT PROTEIN IMPORTANT?

Protein is an important part of any diet. As a child's body uses protein, it produces waste that the kidneys must remove from the blood. Too much protein can cause waste to build up in a child's blood.

However, too little protein can prevent children with CKD from growing normally and obtaining important nutrients. The goal is for children to consume enough protein to grow while avoiding excessive amounts.

Children on Dialysis

Children on dialysis need to eat somewhat more protein because the dialysis treatment removes some protein from the blood. The amount of protein removed from the blood depends on the type of dialysis treatment.

A child's protein needs will change over time. A dietitian can work with parents and the child to adapt meal plans to their changing needs.

WHY IS KNOWING ABOUT SODIUM IMPORTANT?

Sodium is a component of salt. Children with CKD have very different sodium needs. Too little sodium can lead to dehydration and poor weight gain in some children, and too much sodium may cause high blood pressure (HBP) in others. What a child eats and drinks can help control the amount of sodium in their diet.

The amount of sodium a child needs will depend on the type and severity of their CKD, their age, and other factors. Parents may need to either limit or add sodium to a child's diet. It is important to talk with a child's health-care team about how much sodium they should have.

If a child's health-care team suggests lowering the amount of sodium in their diet, parents can help by:

- buying fresh fruits and vegetables
- choosing unprocessed meats instead of processed foods
- cooking from scratch
- using spices, herbs, and salt-free seasonings instead of salt
- looking for products labeled "sodium-free" or "low sodium"
- draining and rinsing canned foods to remove salt

WHY IS KNOWING ABOUT POTASSIUM IMPORTANT?

In some children with CKD, the kidneys do a poor job of removing potassium from the blood, leading to high blood potassium levels. Both too little and too much potassium can cause heart and muscle problems. Children with CKD should have their blood checked regularly to ensure their potassium levels are normal. A child's food and drink choices can affect their potassium level. Parents should talk with a child's health-care team about how much potassium their child should consume.

If the health-care team suggests that a child needs to lower their potassium intake, parents can help by:

- selecting fruits and vegetables that are lower in potassium
- draining canned fruits and vegetables and discarding the liquid, which is often high in potassium
- using spices and herbs instead of salt substitutes, which can be very high in potassium
- consulting with the child's dietitian about choosing foods the child enjoys that have the right amount of potassium

WHY IS KNOWING ABOUT PHOSPHORUS IMPORTANT?

Phosphorus can build up in the blood of children with CKD. Excess phosphorus can weaken a child's bones.

Phosphorus is found naturally in foods rich in protein. It is also added to many processed foods, flavored drinks, and some meats. Phosphorus additives are a primary source of phosphorus for many people with CKD. Phosphorus added to food may cause a child's blood phosphorus levels to rise more than phosphorus found naturally in food. A dietitian can help parents find ways for their child to get enough protein without excessive phosphorus.

As kidney disease progresses, a child may need to take a phosphate binder with meals to lower the amount of phosphorus in the blood. A phosphate binder is a medicine that acts like a sponge to soak up or bind phosphorus while in the stomach. Because it is bound, the phosphorus does not enter the child's blood. Instead, the child's body removes the phosphorus through their stool.

SHOULD YOUR CHILD TAKE VITAMIN AND MINERAL SUPPLEMENTS?

Children with CKD may not get enough of certain vitamins and minerals because they have to limit some foods, or they may not feel hungry and do not eat enough of certain foods. If a child is on dialysis, they may lose water-soluble vitamins during the dialysis treatment.

A child's kidney care specialist may prescribe vitamin And mineral supplements specifically designed for children with kidney failure.

Never give a child vitamin And mineral supplements available over the counter (OTC). OTC vitamin And mineral supplements may be harmful to children with kidney failure. For safety reasons, parents should consult with their child's health-care team before giving any medicines, vitamin And mineral supplements, or probiotics that have not been prescribed for their child.

WHAT ARE SOME SPECIAL PROBLEMS FOR INFANTS WITH CHRONIC KIDNEY DISEASE?

Because infants grow so quickly, the health-care team will need to monitor an infant with CKD closely. Often, infants require special formulas with extra supplements and calories to ensure they receive the right amount of fluid and nutrients. If an infant cannot drink the needed amount of formula, the health-care professional may suggest tube feeding. Tube feeding is often the best way to ensure a child receives the full supply of fluid and nutrients needed for proper growth and development.[1]

[1] "Nutrition for Children with Chronic Kidney Disease," National Institute of Diabetes and Digestive and Kidney Diseases (NIDDK), December 2019. Available online. URL: www.niddk.nih.gov/health-information/kidney-disease/children/helping-child-adapt-life-chronic-kidney-disease/nutrition-chronic-kidney-disease. Accessed October 15, 2024.

Part 2 | Disorders and Diseases of the Kidneys

Chapter 7 | Chronic Kidney Disease

Chapter Contents

Section 7.1 | Understanding Chronic Kidney Disease

WHAT ARE YOUR KIDNEYS?

Your kidneys, each just the size of a computer mouse, filter all the blood in your body every 30 minutes. They work hard to remove wastes, toxins, and excess fluid. They also:

- help control blood pressure
- signal the body to produce red blood cells
- help keep your bones healthy
- regulate blood chemicals that are essential to life

Properly functioning kidneys are critical for maintaining good health.

CHRONIC KIDNEY DISEASE

Chronic kidney disease (CKD) is a condition in which the kidneys are damaged and cannot filter blood as well as they should. Because of this, excess fluid and waste remain in the body, potentially causing health problems such as heart disease.

KIDNEY DISEASE FACTS

- More than one in seven U.S. adults may have CKD.
- As many as 9 in 10 do not know they have it.
- Kidney diseases are a leading cause of death in the United States.
- About 360 people begin treatment for kidney failure (dialysis or kidney transplant) every day.

CHRONIC KIDNEY DISEASE BY THE NUMBERS

- Kidney diseases are a leading cause of death in the United States.
- About 35.5 million U.S. adults are estimated to have CKD, and most are undiagnosed.
- 40 percent of people with severely reduced kidney function (not on dialysis) are not aware of having CKD.

- Every 24 hours, 360 people begin dialysis treatment for kidney failure.
- In the United States, diabetes and high blood pressure (HBP) are the leading causes of kidney failure, accounting for two out of three new cases.
- In 2019, treating Medicare beneficiaries with CKD cost $87.2 billion, and treating people with end-stage kidney disease (ESKD) cost an additional $37.3 billion.

MEDICARE COSTS

In 2019, treatment for Medicare beneficiaries with CKD cost $87.2 billion, and treatment for people with ESKD cost an additional $37.3 billion.

Costs can be reduced by preventing:

- CKD in people at risk.
- CKD from progressing to ESKD.
- Other chronic conditions such as type 2 diabetes and heart disease, which can lead to CKD.

HEALTH PROBLEMS RELATED TO CHRONIC KIDNEY DISEASE

Health problems related to CKD include:

- anemia or a low number of red blood cells
- increased occurrence of infections
- low calcium levels, high potassium levels, and high phosphorus levels in the blood
- loss of appetite or eating less
- depression or lower quality of life

CKD has varying levels of seriousness. It usually worsens over time, though treatment has been shown to slow progression. CKD can progress to kidney failure and early cardiovascular disease.

When the kidneys stop working, dialysis or a kidney transplant is needed for survival. Kidney failure treated with dialysis or kidney transplant is called "end-stage kidney disease." Not all people with kidney disease progress to kidney failure.

SYMPTOMS OF CHRONIC KIDNEY DISEASE

People with CKD may not feel ill or notice any symptoms. The only way to find out for sure if you have CKD is through blood and urine tests. These tests measure both the creatinine level in the blood and protein in the urine.

RISK FACTORS OF CHRONIC KIDNEY DISEASE

Diabetes

Chronic kidney disease is common in people with diabetes. Approximately one in three adults with diabetes has CKD. Each kidney is made up of millions of tiny filters called "nephrons." High blood sugar from diabetes can damage blood vessels in the kidneys and nephrons, preventing them from working properly.

High Blood Pressure

Approximately one in five adults with HBP have CKD. HBP can make blood vessels narrower, reducing blood flow. Over time, blood vessels throughout the body weaken, including those in the kidneys. Damaged blood vessels in the kidneys may no longer function properly. When this happens, the kidneys cannot remove all wastes and extra fluid from the body, which can raise your blood pressure even more.

Heart Disease

Adults with heart failure have a higher risk of CKD due to reduced blood flow to the kidneys. Having CKD is also a risk factor for heart disease.

Family History

Chronic kidney disease tends to run in families. You may be more likely to develop kidney disease if you have a close relative with CKD.

Obesity

Being overweight or obese raises your risk for HBP and diabetes, the two biggest causes of CKD. This means that being overweight or obese puts you at greater risk for CKD.

REDUCING CHRONIC KIDNEY DISEASE RISK

- Keep your blood pressure below 140/90 mm Hg (or the target your doctor sets for you).
- If you have diabetes, stay within your target blood sugar range as much as possible.
- Get active. Physical activity helps control blood pressure and blood sugar levels.
- Lose weight if needed.
- Get tested for CKD regularly if you are at risk.
- If you have CKD, meet with a dietitian to create a kidney-healthy eating plan. The plan may need to change as you get older or if your health status changes.
- Take medicines as instructed and ask your doctor about blood pressure medicines called "angiotensin-converting enzyme inhibitors" and "angiotensin II receptor blockers," which may protect your kidneys in addition to lowering blood pressure.
- If you smoke, make a plan to quit. Smoking can worsen kidney disease and interfere with medication that lowers blood pressure.
- Include a kidney doctor (nephrologist) on your health-care team.[1]

Section 7.2 | Common Causes of Chronic Kidney Disease

Diabetes and high blood pressure (HBP) are the most common causes of chronic kidney disease (CKD). Your health-care provider will review your health history and may perform tests to determine the underlying cause of your kidney disease. The cause of your kidney disease may affect the type of treatment you receive.

[1] "Chronic Kidney Disease Basics," Centers for Disease Control and Prevention (CDC), May 15, 2024. Available online. URL: www.cdc.gov/kidney-disease/about. Accessed October 16, 2024.

DIABETES

Excess glucose, also called "sugar," in your blood damages your kidneys' filters. Over time, your kidneys can become so damaged that they no longer effectively filter wastes and extra fluid from your blood.

Often, the first sign of kidney disease resulting from diabetes is protein in urine. When the filters are damaged, a protein called "albumin," which is necessary for maintaining health, leaks from the blood into the urine. A healthy kidney does not allow albumin to pass from the blood into the urine.

Diabetic kidney disease is the medical term for kidney disease caused by diabetes.

HIGH BLOOD PRESSURE

High blood pressure can damage blood vessels in the kidneys, reducing their ability to function properly. If the blood vessels in your kidneys are damaged, your kidneys may not effectively remove wastes and extra fluid from your body. The accumulation of extra fluid in the blood vessels can raise blood pressure even further, creating a dangerous cycle.

OTHER CAUSES OF KIDNEY DISEASE

Other causes of kidney disease include:

- a genetic disorder that causes many cysts to grow in the kidneys, known as "polycystic kidney disease" (PKD)
- an infection
- a drug that is toxic to the kidneys
- a disease that affects the entire body, such as diabetes or lupus nephritis
- IgA glomerulonephritis
- disorders in which the body's immune system attacks its own cells and organs, such as anti-GBM (Goodpasture) disease
- heavy metal poisoning, such as lead poisoning
- rare genetic conditions, such as Alport syndrome

- hemolytic uremic syndrome in children
- IgA vasculitis
- renal artery stenosis[1]

Section 7.3 | Strategies for Managing Chronic Kidney Disease

If you have chronic kidney disease (CKD), you can take steps to protect your kidneys from further damage. The sooner you know you have kidney disease, the better. Protecting your kidneys from damage may also help prevent heart disease and improve your overall health. Making these changes when you have no symptoms may be challenging, but it is worthwhile.

CONTROL YOUR BLOOD PRESSURE

The most important step you can take to manage kidney disease is to control your blood pressure. High blood pressure (HBP) can damage your kidneys. You can protect your kidneys by keeping your blood pressure at or below the goal set by your health-care provider. For most people, the blood pressure goal is less than 140/90 mm Hg.

Work with your health-care provider to develop a plan to meet your blood pressure goals. Steps you can take to meet your blood pressure goals may include:

- eating heart-healthy and low-sodium meals
- quitting smoking
- being physically active
- getting enough sleep
- taking your medications as prescribed

[1] "Causes of Chronic Kidney Disease," National Institute of Diabetes and Digestive and Kidney Diseases (NIDDK), October 2016. Available online. URL: www.niddk.nih.gov/health-information/kidney-disease/chronic-kidney-disease-ckd/causes. Accessed October 16, 2024.

MEET YOUR BLOOD GLUCOSE GOAL IF YOU HAVE DIABETES

To reach your blood glucose goal, check your blood glucose level regularly. Use the results to guide decisions about food, physical activity, and medications. Ask your health-care provider how often you should check your blood glucose level.

Your health-care provider will also test your A1C. The A1C is a blood test that measures your average blood glucose level over the past three months. This test is different from the blood glucose checks you perform regularly. The higher your A1C number, the higher your blood glucose levels have been during the past three months. Staying close to your daily blood glucose numbers will help you meet your A1C goal.

For many people with diabetes, the A1C goal is below 7 percent. Ask your health-care provider what your goal should be. Reaching your target numbers will help you protect your kidneys.

WORK WITH YOUR HEALTH-CARE TEAM TO MONITOR YOUR KIDNEY HEALTH

The tests that health-care providers use to assess kidney disease can also track changes in kidney function and damage. Kidney disease tends to worsen over time. Each time you undergo testing, ask your provider how the results compare to previous tests. Your goals will be to:

- keep your glomerular filtration rate (GFR) stable
- keep your urine albumin levels the same or lower

Your health-care provider will also check your blood pressure and, if you have diabetes, your A1C level to ensure you are meeting your blood pressure and blood glucose goals.

How Can You Prepare for Visits with Your Health-Care Provider?

The more you plan for your visits, the more you will be able to learn about your health and treatment options.

Make a List of Questions

It is normal to have many questions. Write down your questions as you think of them so that you can remember everything you want to ask when you see your health-care provider. You may want to ask about what tests are being conducted, what the test results mean, or the changes you need to make to your diet and medications.

Bring a Friend or Relative with You for Support

A trusted friend or family member can take notes, ask questions you may not have considered, offer support, and help remember what the provider said during the visit. Discuss ahead of time what you want to achieve from the visit and the role you would like your friend or relative to play.

TAKE MEDICINES AS PRESCRIBED

Many people with CKD take medications prescribed to lower blood pressure, control blood glucose, and reduce cholesterol levels.

Two types of blood pressure medications, angiotensin-converting enzyme (ACE) inhibitors and angiotensin II receptor blockers (ARBs), may slow kidney disease and delay kidney failure, even in people who do not have HBP. The names of these medications typically end in –pril or –sartan.

Many people need to take two or more medications for their blood pressure. You may also need to take a diuretic, sometimes called a "water pill." The aim is to meet your blood pressure goal. These medications may work better if you limit your salt intake.

Tips for Managing Your Medicines

The next time you pick up a prescription or purchase an OTC medication or supplement, ask your pharmacist how the product may:

- affect your kidneys
- interact with other medications you take

Fill your prescriptions at only one pharmacy or pharmacy chain so your pharmacist can:

- keep track of your medications and supplements
- check for harmful interactions

Keep track of your medications and supplements:

- Maintain an up-to-date list of your medications and supplements in your wallet. Bring your list with you, or take all of your medication bottles, to all health-care visits.

WORK WITH A DIETITIAN TO DEVELOP A MEAL PLAN

What you eat and drink can help you:

- protect your kidneys
- achieve your blood pressure and blood glucose goals
- prevent or delay health problems caused by kidney disease

As your kidney disease progresses, you may need to make additional changes to your diet.

A dietitian who specializes in kidney disease can help you create a meal plan that includes foods that are healthy and enjoyable to eat. Cooking and preparing your food from scratch can promote healthier eating.

Nutrition counseling from a registered dietitian to help meet your medical or health goals is called "medical nutrition therapy" (MNT). If you have diabetes or kidney disease and have a referral from your primary care provider, your health insurance may cover MNT. If you qualify for Medicare, MNT is covered.

Your health-care provider may be able to refer you to a dietitian. You can also find a registered dietitian online through the Academy of Nutrition and Dietetics. Work closely with your dietitian to learn to eat properly for CKD.

MAKE PHYSICAL ACTIVITY PART OF YOUR ROUTINE

Be active for 30 minutes or more on most days. Physical activity can help you reduce stress, manage your weight, and achieve your blood pressure and blood glucose goals. If you are not currently active, ask your health-care provider about the types and amounts of physical activity that are appropriate for you.

AIM FOR A HEALTHY WEIGHT

Being overweight makes your kidneys work harder and may damage your kidneys. The National Institutes of Health (NIH) Body Weight Planner is an online tool to help you tailor your calorie and physical activity plans to achieve and maintain a healthy weight.

GET ENOUGH SLEEP

Aim for seven to eight hours of sleep each night. Getting sufficient sleep is important for your overall physical and mental health and can help you meet your blood pressure and blood glucose goals. You can take steps to improve your sleep habits.

STOP SMOKING

Cigarette smoking can exacerbate kidney damage. Quitting smoking may help you meet your blood pressure goals, which is beneficial for your kidneys, and can lower your chances of having a heart attack or stroke.

FIND HEALTHY WAYS TO COPE WITH STRESS AND DEPRESSION

Long-term stress can elevate your blood pressure and blood glucose levels and lead to depression. Some of the steps you are taking to manage your kidney disease are also healthy ways to cope with stress. For example, physical activity and sleep help reduce stress. Listening to your favorite music, focusing on something calm or peaceful, or meditating may also be beneficial.

Depression is common among individuals with a chronic illness. It can make managing your kidney disease more difficult. Seek help if you feel down. Consider consulting a mental health professional. Talking with a support group, clergy member, friend, or family member who will listen to your feelings may also help.[1]

[1] "Managing Chronic Kidney Disease," National Institute of Diabetes and Digestive and Kidney Diseases (NIDDK), October 2016. Available online. URL: www.niddk.nih.gov/health-information/kidney-disease/chronic-kidney-disease-ckd/managing. Accessed October 16, 2024.

Section 7.4 | Preventing Kidney Disease through Healthy Habits

RISK FACTORS FOR KIDNEY DISEASE

You are more likely to develop kidney disease if you have:

- diabetes
- high blood pressure (HBP)
- heart disease
- a family history of kidney failure

WHAT CAN I DO TO KEEP MY KIDNEYS HEALTHY?

You can protect your kidneys by preventing or managing health conditions that cause kidney damage, such as diabetes and HBP. The steps described below may help keep your entire body healthy, including your kidneys.

During your next medical visit, you may want to ask your health-care provider about your kidney health. Early kidney disease may not present any symptoms, so getting tested may be the only way to know your kidneys are healthy. Your health-care provider will help decide how often you should be tested.

See a provider right away if you develop a urinary tract infection (UTI), which can cause kidney damage if left untreated.

Make Healthy Food Choices

Choose foods that are beneficial for your heart and your entire body, including fresh fruits, fresh or frozen vegetables, whole grains, and low-fat or fat-free dairy products. Eat healthy meals and reduce your intake of salt and added sugars. Aim for less than 2,300 milligrams of sodium each day. Strive to have less than 10 percent of your daily calories come from added sugars.

TIPS FOR MAKING HEALTHY FOOD CHOICES

- Cook with a mix of spices instead of salt.
- Choose veggie toppings such as spinach, broccoli, and peppers for your pizza.

- Try baking or broiling meat, chicken, and fish instead of frying.
- Serve foods without gravy or added fats.
- Select foods with little or no added sugar.
- Gradually transition from whole milk to 2 percent milk until you are using fat-free (skim) or low-fat milk and milk products.
- Consume foods made from whole grains—such as whole wheat, brown rice, oats, and whole-grain corn—every day. Use whole-grain bread for toast and sandwiches; substitute brown rice for white rice in home-cooked meals and when dining out.
- Read food labels. Choose foods low in saturated fats, trans fats, cholesterol, salt (sodium), and added sugars.
- Slow down at snack time. Eating a bag of low-fat popcorn takes longer than eating a slice of cake. Peel and eat an orange instead of drinking orange juice.
- Try keeping a written record of your food intake for a week. This can help you identify when you tend to overeat or consume foods high in fat or calories.

Make Physical Activity Part of Your Routine

Be active for 30 minutes or more on most days. If you are not currently active, ask your health-care provider about the types and amounts of physical activity that are right for you. Add more activity to your life with these tips to help you get active.

Aim for a Healthy Weight

If you are overweight or have obesity, work with your health-care provider or dietitian to create a realistic weight-loss plan.

Get Enough Sleep

Aim for seven to eight hours of sleep each night. If you have trouble sleeping, take steps to improve your sleep habits.

Stop Smoking

If you smoke or use other tobacco products, quit. Ask for help so you do not have to do it alone.

Limit Alcohol Intake

Drinking excessive alcohol can raise your blood pressure and add extra calories, which can lead to weight gain. If you consume alcohol, limit yourself to one drink per day if you are a woman and two drinks per day if you are a man. One drink is defined as:

- 12 ounces of beer
- 5 ounces of wine
- 1.5 ounces of liquor

Explore Stress-Reducing Activities

Learning how to manage stress, relax, and cope with problems can improve emotional and physical health. Physical activity, as well as mind-body practices such as meditation, yoga, or tai chi, can help reduce stress.

Manage Diabetes, High Blood Pressure, and Heart Disease

If you have diabetes, HBP, or heart disease, the best way to protect your kidneys from damage includes the following measures:

- **Keep your blood glucose levels close to your target.** Regularly checking your blood glucose—or blood sugar—level is an important way to manage your diabetes. Your health-care team may want you to test your blood glucose one or more times a day.
- **Maintain your blood pressure numbers within the target range.** The blood pressure goal for most people with diabetes is below 140/90 mm Hg.
- **Take all your medications as prescribed.** Discuss with your health-care provider certain blood pressure medications called "angiotensin-converting enzyme (ACE) inhibitors" and "angiotensin II receptor

blockers" (ARBs), which may protect your kidneys. The names of these medications typically end in –pril or –sartan.
- **Be cautious about the daily use of over-the-counter pain medications.** Regular use of nonsteroidal anti-inflammatory drugs (NSAIDs), such as ibuprofen and naproxen, can damage your kidneys.

Keep your cholesterol levels within the target range to help prevent heart attacks and strokes. There are two types of cholesterol in your blood: LDL and HDL. LDL, or "bad" cholesterol, can build up and clog your blood vessels, potentially causing a heart attack or stroke. HDL, or "good" cholesterol, helps remove "bad" cholesterol from your blood vessels. A cholesterol test may also measure another type of blood fat called "triglycerides."

Ask Your Health-Care Provider Questions

Ask your health-care provider the following key questions about your kidney health during your next medical visit. The sooner you know you have kidney disease, the sooner you can receive treatment to help protect your kidneys.

KEY QUESTIONS FOR YOUR HEALTH-CARE PROVIDER

- What is my glomerular filtration rate (GFR)?
- What is my urine albumin result?
- What is my blood pressure?
- What is my blood glucose level (for people with diabetes)?
- How often should I get my kidneys checked?

OTHER IMPORTANT QUESTIONS

- What should I do to keep my kidneys healthy?
- Do I need to take different medications?
- Should I be more physically active?
- What kind of physical activity can I do?
- What can I eat?

Chronic Kidney Disease

- Am I at a healthy weight?
- Do I need to talk with a dietitian to get help with meal planning?
- Should I be taking ACE inhibitors or ARBs for my kidneys?
- What happens if I have kidney disease?[1]

[1] "Preventing Chronic Kidney Disease," National Institute of Diabetes and Digestive and Kidney Diseases (NIDDK), October 2016. Available online. URL: www.niddk.nih.gov/health-information/kidney-disease/chronic-kidney-disease-ckd/prevention. Accessed October 16, 2024.

Chapter 8 | Renal Artery Stenosis

WHAT ARE RENAL ARTERY STENOSIS AND RENOVASCULAR HYPERTENSION?

Renal artery stenosis (RAS) is the narrowing of one or both renal arteries. "Renal" means "kidney," and "stenosis" means "narrowing." The renal arteries are blood vessels that carry blood to the kidneys from the aorta—the main blood vessel that carries blood from the heart to arteries throughout the body (see Figure 8.1).

Renovascular hypertension (RVH) is high blood pressure (HBP) caused by RAS. Blood pressure is expressed with two numbers separated by a slash, 120/80, and is said as "120 over 80." The top number is called the "systolic pressure" and represents the pressure as the heart beats and pushes blood through the blood vessels. The bottom number is called the "diastolic pressure" and represents the pressure as blood vessels relax between heartbeats. A person's blood pressure is considered normal if it remains at or below 120/80. HBP is defined as a systolic pressure of 140 or above or a diastolic pressure of 90 or above.

WHAT CAUSES RENAL ARTERY STENOSIS?

About 90 percent of RAS is caused by atherosclerosis, which is the clogging, narrowing, and hardening of the renal arteries. In these cases, RAS develops when plaque—a sticky substance made up of fat, cholesterol, calcium, and other materials found in the blood—builds up on the inner wall of one or both renal arteries. Plaque buildup makes the artery wall hard and narrow.

Most other cases of RAS are caused by fibromuscular dysplasia (FMD)—the abnormal development or growth of cells on the renal artery walls—which can cause blood vessels to narrow. Rarely, RAS is caused by other conditions.

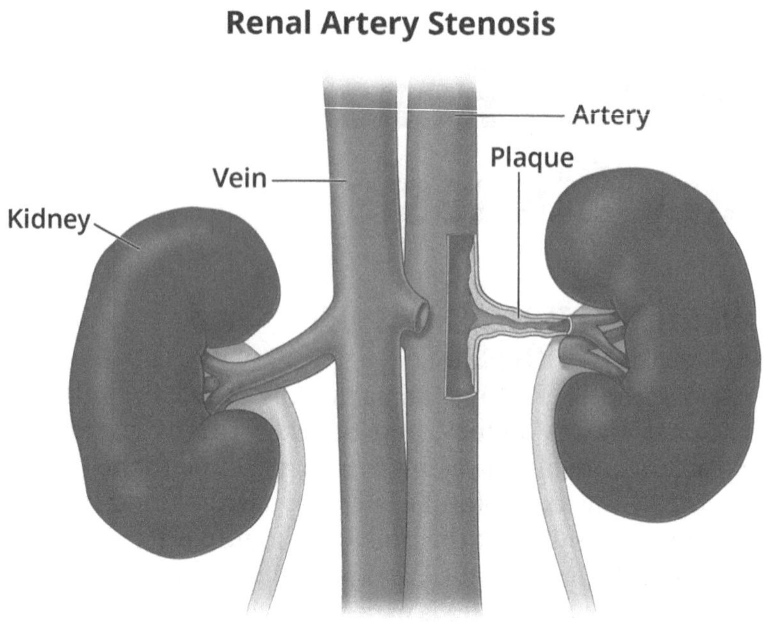

Figure 8.1. Renal Artery Stenosis

National Institute of Diabetes and Digestive and Kidney Diseases (NIDDK)

WHO IS AT RISK FOR RENAL ARTERY STENOSIS?

People at risk for atherosclerosis are also at risk for RAS. Risk factors for RAS caused by atherosclerosis include:

- high blood cholesterol levels
- high blood pressure
- smoking
- insulin resistance
- diabetes
- being overweight or having obesity
- lack of physical activity
- a diet high in fat, cholesterol, sodium, and sugar

- being a man older than 45 or a woman older than 55
- a family history of early heart disease

The risk factors for RAS caused by FMD are unknown, but FMD is most common in women and people aged 25–50. FMD can affect more than one person in a family, indicating that it may be caused by an inherited gene.

WHAT ARE THE SYMPTOMS OF RENAL ARTERY STENOSIS?

In many cases, RAS has no symptoms until it becomes severe.

The signs of RAS are usually either high blood pressure or decreased kidney function—or both—but RAS is often overlooked as a cause of high blood pressure. RAS should be considered as a cause of HBP in people who:

- are older than age 50 when they develop high blood pressure or experience a marked increase in blood pressure
- have no family history of high blood pressure
- cannot be successfully treated with at least three different types of blood pressure medications

Symptoms of a significant decrease in kidney function include:

- increase or decrease in urination
- edema—swelling, usually in the legs, feet, or ankles and less often in the hands or face
- drowsiness or tiredness
- generalized itching or numbness
- dry skin
- headaches
- weight loss
- appetite loss
- nausea
- vomiting
- sleep problems
- trouble concentrating

- darkened skin
- muscle cramps

WHAT ARE THE POSSIBLE COMPLICATIONS OF RENAL ARTERY STENOSIS?

People with RAS are at increased risk for complications resulting from loss of kidney function or atherosclerosis occurring in other blood vessels, such as:

- chronic kidney disease (CKD)—reduced kidney function over a period of time
- coronary artery disease—narrowing and hardening of arteries that supply blood to the heart
- stroke—brain damage caused by a lack of blood flow to the brain
- peripheral vascular disease—blockage of blood vessels that restricts blood flow from the heart to other parts of the body, particularly the legs

RAS can lead to kidney failure, described as "end-stage renal disease" when treated with blood-filtering treatments called "dialysis" or a "kidney transplant," though this is uncommon in people who receive ongoing treatment for RAS.

HOW IS RENAL ARTERY STENOSIS DIAGNOSED?

A health-care provider can diagnose RAS by listening to the abdomen with a stethoscope and performing imaging tests. When blood flows through a narrow artery, it sometimes makes a whooshing sound, called a "bruit." The health-care provider may place a stethoscope on the front or side of the abdomen to listen for this sound. The absence of this sound, however, does not exclude the possibility of RAS.

In some cases, RAS is found when a person has a test for another reason. For example, a health-care provider may discover RAS during a coronary angiogram for the diagnosis of heart problems. A coronary angiogram is a procedure that uses a special dye, called "contrast medium," and x-rays to visualize how blood flows through the heart.

HOW IS RENAL ARTERY STENOSIS TREATED?

Treatment for RAS includes lifestyle changes, medications, and surgery and aims to:

- prevent RAS from worsening
- treat RVH
- relieve the blockage of the renal arteries

RAS that has not led to RVH or caused a significant blockage of the artery may not need treatment. RAS that requires treatment, also called "critical RAS," is defined by the American Heart Association as a reduction of more than 60 percent in the diameter of the renal artery. However, health-care providers are not entirely sure what degree of blockage will cause significant problems.

Lifestyle Changes

The first step in treating RAS is making lifestyle changes that promote healthy blood vessels throughout the body, including the renal arteries. The best ways to prevent plaque buildup in the arteries are to exercise, maintain a healthy body weight, and choose healthy foods. People who smoke should quit to help protect their kidneys and other internal organs.

Medications

People with RVH may need to take medications that—when taken as prescribed by their health-care provider—lower blood pressure and can also significantly slow the progression of kidney disease. Two types of blood pressure-lowering medications, angiotensin-converting enzyme (ACE) inhibitors and angiotensin receptor blockers (ARBs), have proven effective in slowing the progression of kidney disease. Many people require two or more medications to control their blood pressure. In addition to an ACE inhibitor or an ARB, a diuretic—a medication that helps the kidneys remove fluid from the blood—may be prescribed. Beta-blockers, calcium channel blockers, and other blood pressure medications may also be necessary. Some people with RAS cannot take an ACE inhibitor or ARB due to the effects on the kidneys. People with RAS who are prescribed an ACE inhibitor or ARB should have their kidney function checked within a few weeks of starting the medication.

A cholesterol-lowering medication to prevent plaque from building up in the arteries and a blood thinner, such as aspirin, to help the blood flow more easily through the arteries may also be prescribed.

Surgery

Although surgery has been used in the past for the treatment of RAS due to atherosclerosis, recent studies have not shown improved outcomes with surgery compared with medication. However, surgery may be recommended for people with RAS caused by FMD or for those whose RAS does not improve with medication. Different types of surgery for RAS include the following. These procedures are performed in a hospital by a vascular surgeon—a doctor who specializes in repairing blood vessels. Anesthesia is needed.

ANGIOPLASTY AND STENTING

Angioplasty is a procedure in which a catheter is inserted into the renal artery, usually through the groin, similar to a catheter angiogram. For angioplasty, a tiny balloon at the end of the catheter can be inflated to flatten the plaque against the artery wall. A small mesh tube, called a "stent," may then be positioned inside the artery to keep the plaque flattened and the artery open. People with RAS caused by FMD may be successfully treated with angioplasty alone, while angioplasty with stenting has a better outcome for people with RAS caused by atherosclerosis.

ENDARTERECTOMY OR BYPASS SURGERY

In an endarterectomy, the plaque is cleaned out of the artery, leaving the inner lining smooth and clear. To create a bypass, a vein or synthetic tube is used to connect the kidney to the aorta. This new path serves as an alternate route for blood to flow around the blocked artery into the kidney. These procedures are not performed as often as in the past due to a high risk of complications during and after the procedure.[1]

---

[1] "Renal Artery Stenosis," National Institute of Diabetes and Digestive and Kidney Diseases (NIDDK), July 2014. Available online. URL: www.niddk.nih.gov/health-information/kidney-disease/renal-artery-stenosis. Accessed October 16, 2024.

Chapter 9 | Childhood Kidney Disease

WHAT IS KIDNEY DISEASE?

Kidney disease is a condition in which the kidneys are damaged and cannot filter the blood as they should. This damage can cause wastes and fluid to build up in the body. Kidney disease can also lead to other health problems.

Acute kidney injury (AKI) is a sudden decrease in kidney function that usually lasts a short time. Although AKI does not last long, it may cause long-lasting effects even after the underlying problem has been treated. If left untreated, AKI can be life-threatening.

Chronic kidney disease (CKD) develops slowly over a long period—usually months to years. CKD may gradually lead to kidney failure, which means a person will most likely need a kidney transplant or dialysis soon to stay healthier longer. Kidney failure that is treated with a kidney transplant or dialysis is called "end-stage kidney disease" or "ESKD."

HOW COMMON IS KIDNEY DISEASE IN CHILDREN?

Kidney disease is not common in children. Researchers do not know exactly how many children are affected by kidney disease because many children have few or no symptoms in the early stages of the disease.

WHICH CHILDREN ARE MORE LIKELY TO DEVELOP KIDNEY DISEASE?

Chronic kidney disease is more common in male children than in female children. In North America, Black children are two to three times more likely to develop CKD compared with white children.

WHAT ARE THE COMPLICATIONS OF KIDNEY DISEASE IN CHILDREN?

Complications of kidney disease in children may include:

- anemia
- cardiovascular disease or heart disease
- electrolyte imbalances in the blood, especially potassium
- growth problems, especially shorter-than-average height
- high blood pressure (HBP), or hypertension
- infection
- metabolic acidosis
- mineral and bone disorder
- cognitive issues
- urinary incontinence

Kidney disease can also affect children's lives in other ways, causing problems related to behavior, relationships, and self-esteem. Children with CKD may have difficulty concentrating and learning and may develop language and motor skills more slowly than their peers.

WHAT ARE THE SYMPTOMS OF KIDNEY DISEASE IN CHILDREN?

Children in the early stages of kidney disease may have few or no symptoms. As kidney disease progresses, symptoms may include:

- swelling in the feet, legs, hands, or face, called "edema"
- increased or decreased urine output. Some children may need to urinate more often and may wet the bed at night
- foamy urine due to excessive protein in the urine, called "proteinuria"
- pink or cola-colored urine caused by blood in the urine, called "hematuria"

Other symptoms may include:

- decreased appetite
- feeling tired

- fever
- high blood pressure
- itchy skin
- nausea or vomiting
- shortness of breath
- trouble concentrating
- weakness
- weight loss
- stunted growth

Symptoms can vary from child to child, depending on the cause of the kidney disease.

WHAT CAUSES KIDNEY DISEASE IN CHILDREN?

Kidney disease in children can be caused by:

- birth defects
- hereditary diseases
- infection
- nephrotic syndrome
- systemic diseases
- trauma
- urine blockage or reflux

HOW DO HEALTH-CARE PROFESSIONALS DIAGNOSE KIDNEY DISEASE IN CHILDREN?

Health-care professionals use a child's medical and family history and a physical exam to diagnose kidney disease. To confirm the diagnosis, health-care professionals may use one or more of the following tests:

- urine tests, to check how well your child's kidneys are filtering blood and to look for proteins in the urine
- blood tests, to test the glomerular filtration rate and to look for underlying diseases
- imaging tests, to see the size and shape of the kidneys and identify any abnormalities
- kidney biopsy, to check for kidney damage and help identify the cause of the kidney disease
- genetic tests, to look for specific gene mutations

If your child's health-care professional suspects kidney disease, your child may be referred to a pediatric nephrologist—a doctor who specializes in treating kidney disease in children.

HOW DO HEALTH-CARE PROFESSIONALS TREAT KIDNEY DISEASE IN CHILDREN?

Health-care professionals treat kidney disease in children by first addressing or controlling any underlying condition that may be causing the kidney damage. They may perform surgery to correct a blockage in the urinary tract or prescribe antibiotics to treat an infection.

Some children with acute kidney injury may need dialysis—treatment to filter wastes and extra fluids from the blood—for a short time while their kidneys recover.

When a child's kidney disease is chronic, or long-lasting, treatment may slow the progression of the disease, ease symptoms, and manage complications.

Children with CKD are at increased risk for infections. Vaccines help prevent many diseases that can result from infections. Discuss with your child's doctor which vaccines are appropriate for your child. Some children with CKD or certain types of kidney diseases may be eligible for the pneumococcal polysaccharide vaccine (PPSV23), which can prevent some bacterial infections.

HOW DO HEALTH-CARE PROFESSIONALS TREAT COMPLICATIONS OF KIDNEY DISEASE IN CHILDREN?

Health-care professionals manage the complications of kidney disease in children by prescribing medications and suggesting changes to what your child eats and drinks.

Medications

Your child's health-care professional may prescribe:

- angiotensin-converting enzyme (ACE) inhibitors and angiotensin receptor blockers (ARBs) to lower blood pressure and help reduce protein loss
- diuretics to reduce swelling and lower blood pressure by removing excess fluid from the blood

- erythropoiesis-stimulating agents and iron supplements to improve anemia by helping the body make more red blood cells
- corticosteroids or other immunosuppressants to reduce the activity of the immune system and decrease swelling
- phosphate binders to improve bone development and growth by reducing phosphorus levels in the blood
- growth hormone therapy injections to increase growth
- pH-adjusting medications, such as sodium bicarbonate, to lower acid levels in the blood
- antibiotics to help fight infection

Dietary Changes

Your child's health-care professional may suggest dietary changes such as:

- monitoring protein, sodium, potassium, and liquid intake
- limiting phosphorus
- taking vitamin And mineral supplements

Consult with your child's health-care professional before making any changes to your child's diet. Your child's health-care professional may suggest working with a registered dietitian to create an eating plan with the right foods and nutrients in the right amounts for your child to grow properly and stay healthy.

WHAT CAN YOU DO TO KEEP YOUR CHILD'S KIDNEYS HEALTHY?

You can help your child with kidney disease by:

- tracking how much liquid your child consumes and working with your child's health-care team to figure out the right amount of liquid for your child
- following all dietary instructions given by your child's health-care team

- ensuring your child takes all medications as prescribed and informing your child's health-care professional immediately if your child has difficulty taking medications or is experiencing side effects
- consulting with your child's health-care team before giving your child any medications, vitamin And mineral supplements, or probiotics that have not been prescribed for your child[1]

[1] "Kidney Disease in Children," National Institute of Diabetes and Digestive and Kidney Diseases (NIDDK), August 2022. Available online. URL: www.niddk.nih.gov/health-information/kidney-disease/children. Accessed October 16, 2024.

Chapter 10 | **Autoimmune and Immune-Related Kidney Disorders**

Chapter Contents

Section 10.1 | Lupus Nephritis

WHAT IS LUPUS NEPHRITIS?

Lupus nephritis is a type of kidney disease caused by systemic lupus erythematosus (SLE or lupus). Lupus is an autoimmune disease—a disorder in which the body's immune system attacks its own cells and organs. Kidney disease caused by lupus may get worse over time and lead to kidney failure. If the kidneys fail, dialysis or a kidney transplant will be needed to maintain health.

WHO GETS LUPUS?

Lupus is much more common in women than in men and most often strikes during the childbearing years. About 9 out of 10 people who have lupus are women. Lupus is also more common in people of African or Asian background. African Americans and Asian Americans are about two to three times more likely to develop lupus than Caucasians. In the United States, 1 out of every 250 African-American women will develop lupus.

WHAT ARE THE SYMPTOMS OF LUPUS NEPHRITIS?

The symptoms of lupus nephritis may include foamy urine and edema—swelling that occurs when the body has too much fluid, usually in the legs, feet, or ankles but less often in the hands or face. High blood pressure may also develop.

Kidney problems often start at the same time or shortly after lupus symptoms appear and can include:

- joint pain or swelling
- muscle pain
- fever with no known cause
- a red rash, often on the face, across the nose and cheeks, sometimes called a "butterfly rash" because of its shape

WHAT TESTS DO HEALTH-CARE PROFESSIONALS USE TO DIAGNOSE LUPUS NEPHRITIS?

Lupus nephritis is diagnosed through urine and blood tests and a kidney biopsy.

Urine Test

A health-care professional uses a urine sample to look for blood and protein in the urine. The sample is collected in a container in a health-care professional's office or lab. For the test, a nurse or technician places a strip of chemically treated paper, called a "dipstick," into the urine. Patches on the dipstick change color when blood or protein is present. A high level of protein or a high number of red blood cells in the urine indicates kidney damage. The urine will also be examined under a microscope to look for kidney cells.

Blood Test

A blood test is used to check kidney function. The test measures creatinine, a waste product from the normal breakdown of muscles in the body. The kidneys remove creatinine from the blood. Health-care professionals use the amount of creatinine in the blood to estimate the glomerular filtration rate (GFR). As kidney disease progresses, the level of creatinine rises.

Kidney Biopsy

A kidney biopsy is a procedure that involves taking a small piece of kidney tissue for examination under a microscope. A doctor performs the biopsy in a hospital using imaging techniques such as ultrasound or a computed tomography (CT) scan to guide the biopsy needle into the kidney. Health-care professionals numb the area to limit pain and use light sedation to help the patient relax during the procedure.

The kidney tissue is examined in a lab by a pathologist—a doctor who specializes in diagnosing diseases.

A kidney biopsy can:

- confirm a diagnosis of lupus nephritis
- determine the extent of disease progression
- guide treatment

HOW DO DOCTORS TREAT LUPUS NEPHRITIS?

Health-care professionals treat lupus nephritis with medicines that suppress the immune system so it stops attacking and damaging the kidneys. The goals of treatment are to:

- reduce inflammation in the kidneys
- decrease immune system activity

- block the body's immune cells from attacking the kidneys directly or making antibodies that attack the kidneys

Medicines

A health-care professional may prescribe a corticosteroid, usually prednisone, a medicine to suppress the immune system, such as cyclophosphamide or mycophenolate mofetil, and hydroxychloroquine, a medicine for people with SLE.

Lupus nephritis can cause high blood pressure in some people. More than one kind of medicine may be needed to control blood pressure. Blood pressure medicines include:

- ACE inhibitors and ARBs, with drug names that end in –pril or –sartan
- diuretics
- beta-blockers
- calcium channel blockers

ACE inhibitors and ARBs may help protect the kidneys, while diuretics assist the kidneys in removing fluid from the body.

WHAT SHOULD BE EATEN IF LUPUS NEPHRITIS IS PRESENT?

If kidney disease is present, dietary changes may be necessary. Dietitians are nutrition experts who can advise on healthy eating and meal planning. Finding a registered dietitian who can help is essential. Eating the right foods can assist in managing kidney disease. If high blood pressure is present, consuming foods with less sodium (a component of salt) may help lower blood pressure.

WHAT ARE THE COMPLICATIONS OF LUPUS NEPHRITIS?

Treatment is generally effective in controlling lupus nephritis and minimizing complications.

Between 10 and 30 percent of people who have lupus nephritis develop kidney failure.

The most severe form of lupus nephritis, called "diffuse proliferative nephritis," can cause scarring in the kidneys. Scars are permanent, and kidney function often declines as more scars form. Early diagnosis and treatment may help prevent lasting damage.

People with lupus nephritis are at high risk for cancer, primarily B-cell lymphoma—a type of cancer that begins in the cells of the immune system. They are also at high risk for heart and blood vessel problems.[1]

Section 10.2 | **Henoch-Schönlein Purpura**

WHAT IS HENOCH-SCHÖNLEIN PURPURA?

Henoch-Schönlein purpura (HSP) is a disease that causes small blood vessels in the body to become inflamed and leak. The primary symptom is a rash that looks like many small raised bruises. HSP can also affect the kidneys, digestive tract, and joints. HSP can occur at any time in life, but it is most common in children between two and six years of age. Most people recover from HSP completely, though kidney damage is the most likely long-term complication. In adults, HSP can lead to chronic kidney disease (CKD) and kidney failure, described as end-stage renal disease (ESRD) when treated with blood-filtering treatments called "dialysis" or a "kidney transplant."

WHAT ARE THE CAUSES OF HENOCH-SCHÖNLEIN PURPURA?

Henoch-Schönlein purpura is caused by an abnormal immune system response in which the body's immune system attacks the body's own cells and organs. Usually, the immune system makes antibodies, or proteins, to protect the body from foreign substances such as bacteria or viruses. In HSP, these antibodies attack the blood vessels. The factors that cause this immune system response are not known. However, in 30–50 percent of cases, people have an upper respiratory tract infection, such as a cold, before getting HSP. HSP has also been associated with:

- infectious agents such as chickenpox, measles, hepatitis, and HIV viruses

[1] "Lupus and Kidney Disease (Lupus Nephritis)," National Institute of Diabetes and Digestive and Kidney Diseases (NIDDK), January 2017. Available online. URL: www.niddk.nih.gov/health-information/kidney-disease/lupus-nephritis. Accessed October 16, 2024.

- medications
- foods
- insect bites
- exposure to cold weather
- trauma

Genetics may increase the risk of HSP, which has occurred in different members of the same family, including twins.

WHAT ARE THE SYMPTOMS OF HENOCH-SCHÖNLEIN PURPURA?

The symptoms of HSP include the following:

- **Rash**. Leaking blood vessels in the skin causes a rash that looks like bruises or small red dots on the legs, arms, and buttocks. The rash may first look like hives and then change to resemble bruises, and it may spread to the chest, back, and face. The rash does not disappear or turn pale when pressed.
- **Digestive tract problems**. HSP can cause vomiting and abdominal pain, which can range from mild to severe. Blood may also appear in the stool, though severe bleeding is rare.
- **Arthritis**. Pain and swelling can occur in the joints, usually in the knees and ankles and less frequently in the elbows and wrists.
- **Kidney involvement**. Hematuria—blood in the urine—is a common sign that HSP has affected the kidneys. Proteinuria—large amounts of protein in the urine—or the development of high blood pressure (HBP) suggests more severe kidney problems.
- **Other symptoms**. In some cases, boys with HSP develop swelling of the testicles. In rare cases, symptoms affecting the central nervous system, such as seizures, and the lungs, such as pneumonia, have been seen.

Though the rash affects all people with HSP, pain in the joints or abdomen precedes the rash in about one-third of cases by as many as 14 days.

WHAT ARE THE COMPLICATIONS OF HENOCH-SCHÖNLEIN PURPURA?

In children, the risk of kidney damage leading to long-term problems may be as high as 15 percent, but kidney failure affects only about 1 percent of children with HSP. Up to 40 percent of adults with HSP will have CKD or kidney failure within 15 years after diagnosis. A rare complication of HSP is intussusception of the bowel, which includes the small and large intestines. With this condition, a section of the bowel folds into itself like a telescope, causing the bowel to become blocked. Women with a history of HSP who become pregnant are at higher risk for HBP and proteinuria during pregnancy.

HOW IS HENOCH-SCHÖNLEIN PURPURA DIAGNOSED?

A diagnosis of HSP is suspected when a person has the characteristic rash and one of the following:

- abdominal pain
- joint pain
- antibody deposits on the skin
- hematuria or proteinuria

Antibody deposits on the skin can confirm the diagnosis of HSP. These deposits can be detected using a skin biopsy, a procedure that involves taking a piece of skin tissue for examination with a microscope. A skin biopsy is performed by a health-care provider in a hospital with little or no sedation and local anesthetic. The skin tissue is examined in a lab by a pathologist—a doctor who specializes in diagnosing diseases.

A kidney biopsy may also be needed. A kidney biopsy is performed by a health-care provider in a hospital with light sedation and local anesthetic. The health-care provider uses imaging techniques such as ultrasound or a computerized tomography scan to guide the biopsy needle into the organ. The kidney tissue is examined in a lab by a pathologist. The test can confirm the diagnosis and be used to determine the extent of kidney involvement, which will help guide treatment decisions.

Hematuria and proteinuria are detected using urinalysis, which tests a urine sample. The urine sample is collected in a special container in a health-care provider's office or commercial facility and can be tested in the same location or sent to a lab for analysis. For the test, a nurse or technician places a strip of chemically treated paper, called a "dipstick," into the urine sample. Patches on the dipstick change color when blood or protein are present in urine.

HOW IS HENOCH-SCHÖNLEIN PURPURA TREATED?

No specific treatment for HSP exists. The main goal of treatment is to relieve symptoms such as joint pain, abdominal pain, and swelling. People with kidney involvement may receive treatment aimed at preventing long-term kidney disease.

Treatment is rarely required for the rash. Joint pain is often treated with nonsteroidal anti-inflammatory medications, such as aspirin or ibuprofen. Recent research has shown corticosteroids—medications that decrease swelling and reduce the activity of the immune system—to be even more effective in treating joint pain. Corticosteroids are also used to treat abdominal pain.

Though rare, surgery may be needed to treat intussusception or to determine the cause of swollen testicles. HSP that affects the kidneys may be treated with corticosteroid and immunosuppressive medications. Immunosuppressive medications prevent the body from making antibodies. Adults with severe, acute kidney failure are treated with high-dose corticosteroids and immunosuppressive cyclophosphamide (Cytoxan).

People with HSP that causes HBP may need to take medications that—when taken as prescribed by their health-care provider—lower blood pressure and can also significantly slow the progression of kidney disease. Two types of blood pressure-lowering medications, angiotensin-converting enzyme (ACE) inhibitors and angiotensin receptor blockers (ARBs), have proven effective in slowing the progression of kidney disease. Many people require two or more medications to control their blood pressure. In addition to an ACE inhibitor or an ARB, a diuretic—a medication that helps the kidneys remove fluid from the blood—may be prescribed.

Beta-blockers, calcium channel blockers, and other blood pressure medications may also be needed.

Blood and urine tests are used to check the kidney function of people with HSP for at least six months after the main symptoms disappear.[1]

---

[1] "Henoch-Schönlein Purpura," National Institute of Diabetes and Digestive and Kidney Diseases (NIDDK), August 2012. Available online. URL: www.niddk.nih.gov/-/media/Files/Kidney-Disease/HSP_508.pdf. Accessed October 16, 2024.

Chapter 11 | Glomerular Diseases

Chapter Contents

WHAT IS GLOMERULAR DISEASE?

Glomerular disease is a condition that can damage the kidneys. The disease attacks tiny filters in the kidneys, called "glomeruli," where the blood is cleaned. Damaged glomeruli can allow proteins and sometimes red blood cells to leak into the urine. One of the proteins in the blood is albumin. If too much albumin leaks into the urine, fluid can build up in the body, leading to swelling in the face, hands, feet, or legs. In some cases, glomerular disease can also prevent the kidneys from properly removing waste products, causing wastes to build up in the blood (see Figure 11.1).

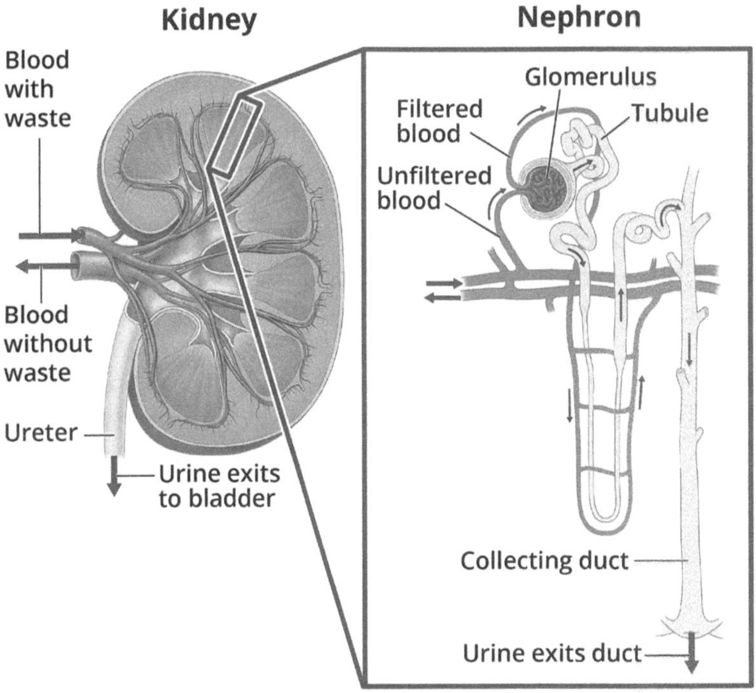

Figure 11.1. Glomeruli Filtering Waste and Retaining Essential Blood Components

National Institute of Diabetes and Digestive and Kidney Diseases (NIDDK)

HOW COMMON IS GLOMERULAR DISEASE?

Most of the diseases that cause glomerular disease are rare. However, one of them, diabetic kidney disease, affects more than one in three U.S. adults who have diabetes. Diabetic kidney disease is also the leading cause of end-stage kidney disease, which is kidney failure that is treated with dialysis or a kidney transplant.

WHO IS MORE LIKELY TO DEVELOP GLOMERULAR DISEASE?

Glomerular disease affects men and women of all ages and all racial and ethnic groups. Having a family member who has glomerular disease increases the risk.

WHAT ARE THE COMPLICATIONS OF GLOMERULAR DISEASE?

Glomerular disease often progresses slowly, causing no symptoms for many years. However, over time, it can cause serious health problems, such as:

- high blood pressure (HBP), also called "hypertension"
- nephrotic syndrome, a group of symptoms that indicate the kidneys are not working properly
- chronic kidney disease, the gradual loss of kidney function, when the kidneys are no longer able to process and remove toxic waste products from the body
- kidney failure, the loss of about 85 percent or more of kidney function, which often leads to symptoms such as appetite loss, nausea, vomiting, and worsening swelling

In some cases, glomerular disease can cause rapid kidney failure that may lead to confusion and death if not treated immediately.

WHAT ARE THE SYMPTOMS OF GLOMERULAR DISEASE?

Symptoms of glomerular disease vary and are related to the type of damage to the glomeruli. Some people with less damage may have few or no symptoms, whereas people with more severe damage may have more noticeable symptoms. Symptoms can include the following:

- **High blood pressure, which may develop or worsen.**
- **Swelling.** Also called "edema," swelling can affect many parts of the body, including the hands, ankles, legs, and around the eyes.
- **Weight gain.** As fluid builds up in the body, weight can increase.
- **Proteinuria.** Too much protein in the urine, called "proteinuria," can cause bubbles or foam to appear in the urine.
- **Blood in the urine.** Also called "hematuria," blood in the urine can make it look pink or cola-colored. The blood can usually only be seen under a microscope.

One or more of these symptoms can be the first sign of kidney disease.

WHAT CAUSES GLOMERULAR DISEASE?

The most common causes of glomerular disease include the following:

- **Diabetic kidney disease, a type of kidney disease caused by diabetes.** Over several years, high levels of blood glucose, also called "blood sugar," can damage the glomeruli.
- **Focal segmental glomerulosclerosis (FSGS), a disease that causes scar tissue to form in some of the kidneys' glomeruli.** FSGS has several causes, including genes, autoimmune diseases, and diseases that cause pressure to build in the glomeruli, such as obesity and sleep apnea.
- **Lupus nephritis, a kidney disease caused by systemic lupus erythematosus (SLE or lupus).** Lupus is an autoimmune disease that affects many parts of the body. The disease can cause antibodies to build up in the glomeruli, causing inflammation that can keep the kidneys from working properly and lead to scarring over time.

- **Membranous nephropathy, a disease that causes antibodies to build up in a part of the kidney called the "glomerular basement membrane."** As a result, the glomeruli can become thick and inflamed. Causes can include infection, cancer, and autoimmune diseases.
- **IgA nephropathy, also called "Berger disease," is an autoimmune disease that causes an antibody called "immunoglobulin A" (IgA) to build up in the glomeruli, causing inflammation and damage.**
- **Minimal change disease, also called "nil disease."** This kidney disease causes changes to the glomeruli that can only be seen under a very powerful microscope, called an "electron microscope."
- **Anti-GBM (Goodpasture) disease, an autoimmune disease in which antibodies attack the glomeruli, causing damage and inflammation.** The disease can also affect the lungs.

Other causes of glomerular disease include:

- infections, including strep throat, bacterial endocarditis, HIV/AIDS, and hepatitis B and C
- some drugs and medicines that can harm the kidneys, such as nonsteroidal anti-inflammatory drugs
- genetic disorders that affect the kidneys, such as Alport syndrome and Fabry disease

In some cases, the exact cause of glomerular disease is unknown.

HOW DO HEALTH-CARE PROFESSIONALS DIAGNOSE GLOMERULAR DISEASE?

Health-care professionals diagnose glomerular disease by ordering tests, such as:

- urinalysis, which examines a sample of urine to find out if levels of protein and red blood cells are too high
- blood tests, which can measure the levels of products in the blood, such as creatinine, urea nitrogen, and a protein called "cystatin C," to find out how well the kidneys are working

- imaging tests, such as an ultrasound or computed tomography (CT) scan, which can show the shape or size of the kidneys
- kidney biopsy, in which a health-care professional examines a small piece of tissue from the kidney under a microscope to look for signs of kidney damage

HOW DO HEALTH-CARE PROFESSIONALS TREAT GLOMERULAR DISEASE?

Treatment for glomerular disease varies based on symptoms, causes, and the extent of kidney damage. In some cases, glomerular disease may resolve once its cause has been treated. In other cases, the disease may go away but later return. Less often, glomerular disease may not respond to treatment and lead to kidney failure over time.

Medicines

Health-care professionals often treat glomerular disease with medicines, such as:

- an angiotensin-converting enzyme (ACE) inhibitor or an angiotensin II receptor blocker (ARB), which can reduce protein loss, lower blood pressure, and slow the progression of kidney disease
- diuretics (water pills), which reduce swelling by helping the kidneys remove sodium—or salt—and water from the blood
- statins, which lower blood cholesterol and can reduce the risk for certain types of heart disease that can develop among people with glomerular disease
- sodium-glucose transporter 2 (SGLT2) inhibitors, medicines originally used to treat diabetes, which can also slow the progression of kidney disease
- medicines that suppress the immune system, such as corticosteroids, antimetabolites, alkylating agents, or monoclonal antibodies, which can reduce inflammation

Other Treatments

If kidney disease advances to kidney failure, health-care professionals may suggest treatment options such as:

- hemodialysis, a procedure that filters blood outside of the body using an external filter called a "dialyzer"
- peritoneal dialysis, a procedure that filters blood inside the body using the lining of the abdomen
- kidney transplant, a surgery that places a healthy kidney from another person inside the body

HOW DO EATING, DIET, AND NUTRITION AFFECT GLOMERULAR DISEASE?

Eating, diet, and nutrition have not been shown to play a role in causing or preventing glomerular disease. However, if one has glomerular disease, health-care professionals may recommend limiting sodium intake, reducing calories if advised to lose excess weight, and limiting saturated fats if cholesterol levels are high.

Understanding glomerular disease, its symptoms, and its implications can aid in timely diagnosis and treatment. Awareness and management can significantly enhance the quality of life for affected individuals.[1]

Section 11.2 | **Nephrotic Syndrome in Adults**

WHAT IS NEPHROTIC SYNDROME?

A nephrotic syndrome is a group of symptoms that indicate your kidneys are not working properly. These symptoms include:

- too much protein in your urine, called "proteinuria"
- low levels of a protein called "albumin" in your blood, called "hypoalbuminemia"

[1] "Glomerular Disease," National Institute of Diabetes and Digestive and Kidney Diseases (NIDDK), June 2022. Available online. URL: www.niddk.nih.gov/health-information/kidney-disease/glomerular-diseases. Accessed October 16, 2024.

- swelling in parts of your body, called "edema"
- high levels of cholesterol and other lipids (fats) in your blood, called "hyperlipidemia"

Your kidneys are made up of about a million filtering units called "nephrons." Each nephron includes a filter, called the "glomerulus," and a tubule. The glomerulus filters your blood, and the tubule returns needed substances to your blood and removes wastes and extra water, which become urine. The nephrotic syndrome usually happens when the glomeruli are inflamed, allowing too much protein to leak from your blood into your urine.

HOW COMMON IS NEPHROTIC SYNDROME?

Nephrotic syndrome is a combination of symptoms that can occur due to different causes. Among adults, the syndrome is most often caused by rare kidney diseases.

WHO IS MORE LIKELY TO DEVELOP NEPHROTIC SYNDROME?

Nephrotic syndrome can affect children and adults of all ages.

WHAT ARE THE COMPLICATIONS OF HAVING NEPHROTIC SYNDROME?

Nephrotic syndrome can lead to serious complications, including:

- blood clots that can lead to thrombosis
- higher risk of infection caused by the loss of immunoglobulins, proteins in your blood that help fight viruses and bacteria
- high blood pressure, also called "hypertension"
- brief or long-lasting kidney problems, including chronic kidney disease and kidney failure

WHAT ARE THE SYMPTOMS OF NEPHROTIC SYNDROME?

Symptoms of nephrotic syndrome can include:

- puffy eyelids and swelling in the legs, ankles, feet, lower abdomen, or other parts of your body
- foamy urine

- weight gain due to retaining too much fluid
- tiredness
- loss of appetite

WHAT CAUSES NEPHROTIC SYNDROME?

Many disorders can cause nephrotic syndrome, including diseases that affect only the kidneys and diseases that affect many parts of the body, such as diabetes and lupus.

Kidney Diseases

Diseases that affect only the kidneys and lead to nephrotic syndrome are called "primary causes" of nephrotic syndrome. The most common primary causes of nephrotic syndrome are as follows:

- **Focal segmental glomerulosclerosis (FSGS).** This disease affects the kidney's glomeruli, causing some of these filters to become scarred. FSGS is the most common cause of nephrotic syndrome in Black adults.
- **Membranous nephropathy.** This disease causes protein to build up in a part of the kidney called the "glomerular basement membrane." It is the most common cause of nephrotic syndrome in white adults.
- **Minimal change disease, also called "nil disease."** This disease is the main cause of nephrotic syndrome in children. Among adults, nephrotic syndrome is more common in older age.

Other Causes

Other causes of nephrotic syndrome, also called "secondary causes," include:

- diabetes
- lupus
- amyloidosis
- infections, such as HIV/AIDS and hepatitis B and C
- some allergic reactions

- some medicines, such as nonsteroidal anti-inflammatory drugs
- genetic disorders that affect the kidneys

In some cases, the exact cause of nephrotic syndrome is unknown.

HOW DO HEALTH-CARE PROFESSIONALS DIAGNOSE NEPHROTIC SYNDROME?

Health-care professionals can diagnose nephrotic syndrome through urine tests. The urine tests show that you are losing too much protein in your urine.

Tests for Diagnosing Nephrotic Syndrome

- **Urine dipstick test.** This simple test checks for albumin in your urine. Having albumin in the urine is called "albuminuria." You collect the urine sample in a container during a visit to a health-care professional's office or lab. A health-care professional places a strip of chemically treated paper, called a "dipstick," into the urine for the test. The dipstick changes color if albumin is present in the urine.

To confirm the diagnosis of nephrotic syndrome, your health-care professional may order one of these two urine tests:

- **24-hour urine collection.** For this test, you will need to collect urine samples over 24 hours. Your health-care professional will then send the samples to a lab for analysis.
- **Urine albumin-to-creatinine ratio (UACR).** The UACR test uses a single urine sample to estimate the amount of albumin lost in 24 hours. The test measures both albumin and creatinine, a waste product of normal muscle breakdown.

Your health-care professional may also order blood tests to check for low protein levels in your blood and other problems linked to nephrotic syndrome.

Tests for Identifying the Cause

Once nephrotic syndrome has been diagnosed, your health-care professional will use tests to identify what caused it and check your kidney function. Tests for finding the cause of nephrotic syndrome can include:

- blood tests
- imaging tests, such as a kidney ultrasound
- kidney biopsy

HOW DO HEALTH-CARE PROFESSIONALS TREAT NEPHROTIC SYNDROME?

Treating Symptoms and Complications

Treatment varies according to symptoms, causes, and the extent of kidney damage. Symptoms of nephrotic syndrome are most often treated with these medicines:

- an angiotensin-converting enzyme (ACE) inhibitor or an angiotensin II receptor blocker (ARB)
- a diuretic (water pill), which reduces swelling by helping the kidneys remove fluid from the blood

In some cases, your health-care professional may also prescribe medicines that lower cholesterol, called "statins." Blood thinners may also be used, but usually only if you develop a blood clot.

To prevent viral and bacterial infections, people with nephrotic syndrome should receive the pneumococcal vaccine and yearly flu shots.

Treating Underlying Causes

Other treatments vary, depending on underlying causes. In some cases, you may need to take medicines that suppress your immune system.

Once the cause has been treated, nephrotic syndrome may disappear, and kidney function may return to normal. Some patients may experience periods of remission followed by times when symptoms reappear. In some cases, nephrotic syndrome may lead to kidney failure.

HOW DO EATING, DIET, AND NUTRITION AFFECT NEPHROTIC SYNDROME?

Eating, diet, and nutrition have not been shown to play a role in causing or preventing nephrotic syndrome. However, if you have developed nephrotic syndrome, your health-care professional may recommend that you take the following actions:

- Limit intake of sodium (salt) and fluids to help control swelling.
- Reduce the amount of fat and cholesterol in your diet to help control your blood cholesterol levels.[1]

Section 11.3 | **Nephrotic Syndrome in Children**

WHAT IS NEPHROTIC SYNDROME?

A nephrotic syndrome is a group of symptoms that indicate the kidneys are not working properly. These symptoms include:

- too much protein in the urine, called "proteinuria"
- low levels of a protein called "albumin" in the blood, called "hypoalbuminemia"
- swelling in parts of the body, called "edema"
- high levels of cholesterol and other lipids (fats) in the blood, called "hyperlipidemia"

The kidneys are made up of about a million filtering units called "nephrons." Each nephron includes a filter, called the "glomerulus," and a tubule. The glomerulus filters the blood, and the tubule returns needed substances to the blood and removes wastes and extra water, which become urine. The nephrotic syndrome usually happens when the glomeruli are damaged, allowing too much protein to leak from the blood into the urine.

[1] "Nephrotic Syndrome in Adults," National Institute of Diabetes and Digestive and Kidney Diseases (NIDDK), October 2020. Available online. URL: www.niddk.nih.gov/health-information/kidney-disease/nephrotic-syndrome-adults. Accessed October 16, 2024.

DOES NEPHROTIC SYNDROME IN CHILDREN HAVE ANOTHER NAME?

Health-care professionals use different terms to refer to nephrotic syndrome in children, depending on:

- how old the child is when symptoms begin
  - congenital nephrotic syndrome: birth to 3 months
  - infantile nephrotic syndrome: 3–12 months
  - childhood nephrotic syndrome: 12 months or older
- the cause of nephrotic syndrome
  - **Primary nephrotic syndrome**. The syndrome is caused by a kidney disease that affects only the kidneys.
  - **Secondary nephrotic syndrome**. The syndrome develops because of other causes, such as diseases that affect other parts of the body, infections, and medicines.

HOW COMMON IS NEPHROTIC SYNDROME IN CHILDREN?

Nephrotic syndrome is not very common in children. On average, fewer than 5 in 100,000 children worldwide develop nephrotic syndrome each year.

WHICH CHILDREN ARE MORE LIKELY TO DEVELOP NEPHROTIC SYNDROME?

Children of all ages can develop nephrotic syndrome. But the condition most often affects children who are two to seven years old, particularly boys.

WHAT ARE THE COMPLICATIONS OF NEPHROTIC SYNDROME IN CHILDREN?

Losing too much protein in the urine can lead to many complications, including:

- higher risk of infection
- blood clots
- high blood pressure (HBP), also called "hypertension"

- high cholesterol
- brief or long-lasting kidney problems

WHAT ARE THE SIGNS OR SYMPTOMS OF NEPHROTIC SYNDROME IN CHILDREN?

Swelling around the eyes is the most common sign of nephrotic syndrome in children. The swelling is usually greater in the morning and, when mild, may be confused with seasonal allergies. Other common symptoms include:

- swelling in the lower legs, feet, abdomen, hands, face, or other parts of the body
- foamy urine
- fatigue

Some children with nephrotic syndrome may also have:

- blood in their urine
- loss of appetite
- muscle cramps
- diarrhea or nausea

WHAT CAUSES NEPHROTIC SYNDROME IN CHILDREN?

Kidney disease that affects a kidney's filtering system is the most common cause of nephrotic syndrome in children. Other causes can include diseases that affect other parts of the body, infections, some medicines, and genetics.

Primary Nephrotic Syndrome

Four ways of kidney disease can cause primary nephrotic syndrome in children and adolescents:

- **Minimal change disease (MCD).** MCD is the most common cause of nephrotic syndrome in young children. The disease causes very little change to the glomeruli or nearby kidney tissue. The changes in the kidney can only be seen using an electron microscope, which shows tiny details. Although the cause of MCD is unknown, some health-care professionals think the immune system may be involved.

- **Focal segmental glomerulosclerosis (FSGS).** This disease can cause some of the kidney's glomeruli to become scarred. FSGS may be caused by genetic variants, or changes in genes present at birth.
- **Membranous nephropathy (MN).** MN is an autoimmune disease that causes immune proteins to build up in the kidney's glomerular basement membrane. As a result, the membrane becomes thick and does not work properly, allowing too much protein to pass into the urine.
- **Other causes of primary nephrotic syndrome are uncommon.**

Secondary Nephrotic Syndrome

Causes of secondary nephrotic syndrome in children include:

- diseases that involve many organs or the whole body, called "systemic diseases"
- infections, including hepatitis B and C, HIV, and malaria
- diseases of the blood, such as leukemia, lymphoma, and sickle cell disease
- some medicines and drugs, such as nonsteroidal anti-inflammatory drugs, and some medicines used to treat mood disorders, bone loss, or cancer

Congenital Nephrotic Syndrome

Among newborns and infants younger than 12 months old, the two most common causes of nephrotic syndrome are:

- genetic variants, which account for most cases of congenital nephrotic syndrome
- infections present at or before birth, such as syphilis and toxoplasmosis

HOW DO HEALTH-CARE PROFESSIONALS DIAGNOSE NEPHROTIC SYNDROME IN CHILDREN?

Nephrotic syndrome in children is diagnosed with:

- a medical and family history
- a physical exam

- urine tests, to look for excess urine proteins
- blood tests, to test kidney function and to look for underlying diseases

Additional tests to identify the cause of nephrotic syndrome may include:

- ultrasound of the kidney
- kidney biopsy
- genetic testing

Many children with nephrotic syndrome will not need a kidney biopsy. The test is usually reserved for children who have complex disease, who have low kidney function, or who are 12 years old or older.

HOW DO HEALTH-CARE PROFESSIONALS TREAT NEPHROTIC SYNDROME IN CHILDREN?

Nephrotic syndrome in children is most often treated with medicines, particularly corticosteroids.

Primary Nephrotic Syndrome

CORTICOSTEROIDS

Corticosteroids, or steroids, are the medicines most often used to treat children with primary nephrotic syndrome. These medicines suppress the immune system, reduce the amount of protein passed into the urine, and decrease swelling.

In most children, treatment with corticosteroids will make nephrotic syndrome improve—also called "remission." If symptoms return, called a "relapse," the health-care professional may prescribe a shorter course of corticosteroids until the disease goes into remission again. Although children may have multiple relapses, they often recover without long-term kidney damage. In most cases, relapses happen less often as children get older.

Although corticosteroids effectively treat nephrotic syndrome in many children, using these medicines for long periods can cause side effects, such as impaired growth, obesity, HBP, eye problems, and bone loss. Other common side effects include anxiety, depression, and aggressive behavior. These problems are more likely to develop with larger doses and longer use.

In some cases, nephrotic syndrome may not improve with corticosteroids. Cases of nephrotic syndrome that do not respond to corticosteroids are more difficult to treat than those that do. They are also more likely to progress to end-stage kidney disease.

OTHER MEDICINES THAT SUPPRESS THE IMMUNE SYSTEM

If corticosteroids are not working or are causing harmful side effects, your child's health-care professional may prescribe other medicines that reduce the activity of the immune system. In some cases, your child may take these medicines together with low-dose corticosteroids.

MEDICINES FOR MANAGING SYMPTOMS AND COMPLICATIONS

Health-care professionals may also prescribe other medicines to help your child manage the symptoms and complications of nephrotic syndrome. Examples include:

- angiotensin-converting enzyme (ACE) inhibitors or angiotensin receptor blockers (ARBs) to lower blood pressure and help reduce protein loss
- diuretics, or water pills, to reduce swelling by helping the kidneys remove extra fluid from the blood
- statins to lower cholesterol
- blood thinners to treat blood clots

Children with nephrotic syndrome should receive the pneumococcal vaccine and yearly flu shots to prevent viral and bacterial infections. They should also get age-appropriate vaccinations. However, the health-care professional may delay certain "live" vaccines—vaccines that use weakened forms of a virus—while your child is taking certain medicines.

Secondary Nephrotic Syndrome

Treatment focuses on the cause of nephrotic syndrome. For example, the health-care professional may:

- prescribe antibiotics to treat an infection that may be causing nephrotic syndrome

- change or stop any medicines your child takes that can cause nephrotic syndrome or make it worse, such as some medicines used to treat lupus, HIV, or diabetes

Your child's health-care professional may also prescribe the same medicines used to manage the symptoms and complications of primary nephrotic syndrome.

Congenital Nephrotic Syndrome

Treatment varies depending on whether the cause is genetic or an infection.

GENETIC

Your child's treatment will depend on the type of genetic mutation that is causing nephrotic syndrome and how severe the symptoms and complications are. Many children will lose kidney function over time and ultimately need a kidney transplant. To keep your child healthy until the transplant, the health-care professional may recommend:

- albumin injections to make up for the albumin passed in urine
- medicines to reduce swelling, lower blood pressure, and reduce protein loss
- removal of one or both kidneys to decrease the loss of albumin in the urine
- dialysis to filter wastes from the blood if the kidneys fail or if both kidneys are removed

INFECTION

When the nephrotic syndrome is caused by a congenital infection, such as syphilis or toxoplasmosis, it will usually resolve when the infection is treated.

HOW CAN NEPHROTIC SYNDROME IN CHILDREN BE PREVENTED?

Researchers have not found a way to prevent nephrotic syndrome in children. Knowing the symptoms can help you get your child treated early and reduce the risk of complications.

HOW DO EATING, DIET, AND NUTRITION AFFECT NEPHROTIC SYNDROME IN CHILDREN?

Children who have nephrotic syndrome may need to change what they eat and drink, such as:

- limiting the amount of sodium they consume, often from salt
- reducing the amount of liquid they drink
- eating foods low in saturated fat and cholesterol

In some cases, the child's health-care professional may recommend other dietary changes. Parents or other caregivers should talk with their child's health-care professional before making any changes to the child's diet.[1]

Section 11.4 | Immunoglobulin A Nephropathy

WHAT IS IMMUNOGLOBULIN A NEPHROPATHY?

Immunoglobulin A (IgA) nephropathy, also known as "Berger disease," is an autoimmune disease that occurs when clumps of antibodies are deposited in the kidneys, causing inflammation and kidney damage. Clumps of immunoglobulin A (IgA) and other antibodies damage the glomeruli, tiny blood vessels in the kidneys that filter blood, causing the kidneys to leak blood and protein into the urine. The damage may also lead to the scarring of the nephrons, the filtering units where the glomeruli are located.

HOW COMMON IS IMMUNOGLOBULIN A NEPHROPATHY?

Immunoglobulin A nephropathy is a common kidney disease and an important cause of chronic kidney disease and kidney failure. About 1 in 10 kidney biopsies in the United States show IgA nephropathy.

[1] "Nephrotic Syndrome in Children," National Institute of Diabetes and Digestive and Kidney Diseases (NIDDK), October 2021. Available online. URL: www.niddk.nih.gov/health-information/kidney-disease/children/childhood-nephrotic-syndrome. Accessed October 16, 2024.

WHO IS MORE LIKELY TO HAVE IMMUNOGLOBULIN A NEPHROPATHY?

Immunoglobulin A nephropathy is more common in people who:

- have a family history of the disease or of IgA vasculitis
- have certain health conditions, such as:
  - celiac disease
  - hepatitis
  - cirrhosis
  - HIV infection
- are aged 10–40
- are of East Asian or white European ancestry
- are male

WHAT ARE THE COMPLICATIONS OF IMMUNOGLOBULIN A NEPHROPATHY?

Complications of IgA nephropathy can include the following:

- **High blood pressure (HBP), also called "hypertension."** Damage to the kidneys caused by IgA nephropathy can increase blood pressure. HBP can further damage the kidneys.
- **Chronic kidney disease.** The slow loss of kidney function over many years can lead to heart disease or stroke.
- **A nephrotic syndrome.** A group of symptoms that point to kidney damage, including high urine protein levels, low blood protein levels, and high levels of cholesterol and other lipids (fats) in the blood, called "hyperlipidemia."
- **Kidney failure.** It occurs when the kidneys do not work well enough to support the body's needs. It can be sudden and temporary—called "acute kidney failure"—or develop over a long time and be permanent. About one in five people with IgA nephropathy develop kidney failure within 10 years of diagnosis.

WHAT ARE THE SYMPTOMS OF IMMUNOGLOBULIN A NEPHROPATHY?

Symptoms can vary and may not appear for years or even decades. Common signs and symptoms include:

- pink or cola-colored urine due to blood in the urine, called "gross hematuria" or "visible hematuria"
- foamy urine from protein leaking into the urine, called "proteinuria"
- swelling due to extra fluid in the legs, feet, ankles, or other parts of the body, called "edema"

WHAT CAUSES IMMUNOGLOBULIN A NEPHROPATHY?

The cause of IgA nephropathy is unknown, but research suggests that genes and the environment may play a role. In some people, the first signs or symptoms of the disease may become noticeable after a cold, sore throat, or other respiratory infection.

HOW DO HEALTH-CARE PROFESSIONALS DIAGNOSE IMMUNOGLOBULIN A NEPHROPATHY?

The health-care professional will conduct a physical exam, review the symptoms and family history, and order urine and blood tests to determine the health of the kidneys.

To make a diagnosis, the health-care professional will order a kidney biopsy. The biopsy can provide valuable information and serve several purposes, including the following:

- Show IgA deposits in the glomeruli.
- Indicate the amount of damage to the kidneys.
- Help predict how the disease will affect the kidneys.
- Help guide treatment.

HOW DO HEALTH-CARE PROFESSIONALS TREAT IMMUNOGLOBULIN A NEPHROPATHY?

Health-care professionals—in most cases, kidney experts called "nephrologists"—treat IgA nephropathy with:

- medicines that help reduce blood pressure and loss of protein in the urine, such as angiotensin-converting

enzyme (ACE) inhibitors or angiotensin receptor blockers (ARB)
- medicines that lower cholesterol and help prevent heart disease, called "statins"
- lifestyle changes, such as limiting sodium (salt) in the diet and quitting smoking

In some cases, the health-care professional may also prescribe immunosuppressants, including corticosteroids. However, these medicines can cause serious side effects, such as weight gain or a weakened immune system.

Although researchers have not yet found a cure for IgA nephropathy, treatment can help prevent or delay damage to the kidneys. New treatments are under development, and several are being evaluated in clinical trials.

In many cases, IgA nephropathy does not get worse over time. However, if the disease progresses to kidney failure, you may need a kidney transplant or blood-filtering treatment called "dialysis."

HOW DO EATING, DIET, AND NUTRITION AFFECT IMMUNOGLOBULIN A NEPHROPATHY?

Researchers have not found evidence that eating, diet, and nutrition play a role in causing or preventing IgA nephropathy. If you have IgA nephropathy, limiting the amount of salt in the diet may help reduce swelling and lower blood pressure. The health-care professional may suggest other changes to the diet based on the symptoms, lab test results, and personal needs.[1]

[1] "IgA Nephropathy," National Institute of Diabetes and Digestive and Kidney Diseases (NIDDK), September 2022. Available online. URL: www.niddk.nih.gov/health-information/kidney-disease/iga-nephropathy. Accessed October 19, 2024.

Section 11.5 | **Goodpasture Syndrome**

WHAT IS GOODPASTURE SYNDROME?

Goodpasture syndrome is a pulmonary-renal syndrome, which is a group of acute illnesses involving the kidneys and lungs. The Goodpasture syndrome includes all the following conditions:

- glomerulonephritis—inflammation of the glomeruli, which are tiny clusters of looping blood vessels in the kidneys that help filter wastes and extra water from the blood
- the presence of anti-glomerular basement membrane (GBM) antibodies; the GBM is part of the glomeruli and is composed of collagen and other proteins
- bleeding in the lungs

In Goodpasture syndrome, immune cells produce antibodies against a specific region of collagen. The antibodies attack the collagen in the lungs and kidneys. Ernest Goodpasture first described the syndrome during the influenza pandemic of 1919 when he reported on a patient who died from bleeding in the lungs and kidney failure. Diagnostic tools to confirm Goodpasture syndrome were not available at that time, so it is not known whether the patient had true Goodpasture syndrome or vasculitis. Vasculitis is an autoimmune condition—a disorder in which the body's immune system attacks the body's own cells and organs—that involves inflammation in the blood vessels and can cause similar lung and kidney problems.

Goodpasture syndrome is sometimes called "anti-GBM disease." However, "anti-GBM disease" is only one cause of pulmonary-renal syndromes, including Goodpasture syndrome. Goodpasture syndrome is fatal unless quickly diagnosed and treated.

WHAT CAUSES GOODPASTURE SYNDROME?

The causes of Goodpasture syndrome are not fully understood. People who smoke or use hair dyes appear to be at increased risk for this condition. Exposure to hydrocarbon fumes, metallic dust, and certain drugs, such as cocaine, may also raise a person's risk.

Genetics may also play a part, as some cases have been reported in more than one family member.

WHAT ARE THE SYMPTOMS OF GOODPASTURE SYNDROME?

The symptoms of Goodpasture syndrome may initially include fatigue, nausea, vomiting, and weakness. The lungs are usually affected before or at the same time as the kidneys, and symptoms can include shortness of breath and coughing, sometimes with blood. The progression from initial symptoms to the lungs being affected may be very rapid. Symptoms that occur when the kidneys are affected include blood in the urine or foamy urine, swelling in the legs, and high blood pressure (HBP).

HOW IS GOODPASTURE SYNDROME DIAGNOSED?

A health-care provider may order the following tests to diagnose Goodpasture syndrome:

- **Urinalysis**. Urinalysis is testing of a urine sample. The urine sample is collected in a special container in a health-care provider's office or commercial facility and can be tested in the same location or sent to a lab for analysis. For the test, a nurse or technician places a strip of chemically treated paper, called a "dipstick," into the urine. Patches on the dipstick change color when protein or blood are present in urine. A high number of red blood cells and high levels of protein in the urine indicate kidney damage.
- **Blood test**. A blood test involves drawing blood at a health-care provider's office or commercial facility and sending the sample to a lab for analysis. It can show the presence of anti-GBM antibodies.
- **Chest x-ray**. An x-ray of the chest is performed in a health-care provider's office, outpatient center, or hospital by an x-ray technician, and the images are interpreted by a radiologist—a doctor who specializes in medical imaging. Abnormalities in the lungs, if present, can be seen on the x-ray.
- **Biopsy**. A biopsy is a procedure that involves taking a piece of kidney tissue for examination with a microscope.

The biopsy is performed by a health-care provider in a hospital with light sedation and local anesthetic. The health-care provider uses imaging techniques such as ultrasound or a computerized tomography scan to guide the biopsy needle into the kidney. The tissue is examined in a lab by a pathologist—a doctor who specializes in diagnosing diseases. The test can show crescent-shaped changes in the glomeruli and lines of antibodies attached to the GBM.

HOW IS GOODPASTURE SYNDROME TREATED?

Goodpasture syndrome is usually treated with:

- immunosuppressive medications, such as cyclophosphamide, to keep the immune system from making antibodies
- corticosteroid medications to suppress the body's autoimmune response
- plasmapheresis—a procedure that uses a machine to remove blood from the body, separate certain cells from the plasma, and return just the cells to the person's body

Plasmapheresis is usually continued for several weeks, and immunosuppressive medications may be given for 6–12 months, depending on the response to therapy. In most cases, bleeding in the lungs stops, and no permanent lung damage occurs. Damage to the kidneys, however, may be long-lasting. If the kidneys fail, blood-filtering treatments called "dialysis" or "kidney transplantation" may become necessary.

EATING, DIET, AND NUTRITION

Eating, diet, and nutrition have not been shown to play a role in causing or preventing Goodpasture syndrome.[1]

[1] "Goodpasture Syndrome," National Institute of Diabetes and Digestive and Kidney Diseases (NIDDK), April 2012. Available online. URL: www.niddk.nih.gov/-/media/Files/Kidney-Disease/GoodpastureSyndrome_508.pdf. Accessed October 19, 2024.

Chapter 12 | Genetic and Congenital Kidney Disorders

Chapter Contents

WHAT IS POLYCYSTIC KIDNEY DISEASE?

Polycystic kidney disease (PKD) is a genetic disorder that causes many fluid-filled cysts to grow in the kidneys (see Figure 12.1). Unlike the usually harmless simple kidney cysts that can form later in life, PKD cysts can change the shape of the kidneys, including making them much larger.

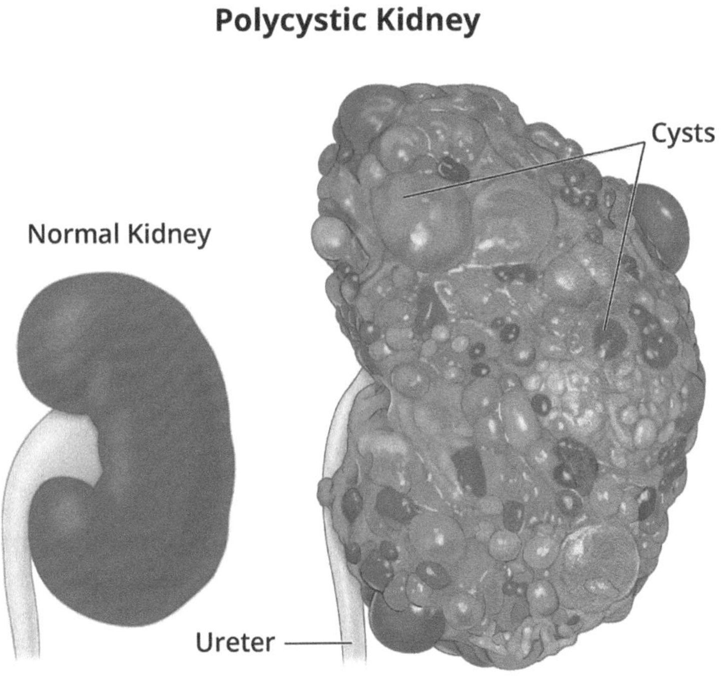

Figure 12.1. Kidneys Affected by Polycystic Kidney Disease

National Institute of Diabetes and Digestive and Kidney Diseases (NIDDK)

PKD is a form of chronic kidney disease (CKD) that reduces kidney function and may lead to kidney failure. PKD also can cause other complications, or problems, such as high blood pressure (HBP), cysts in the liver, and problems with blood vessels in your brain and heart.

WHAT ARE THE TYPES OF POLYCYSTIC KIDNEY DISEASE?

The two main types of PKD are:

- **Autosomal dominant PKD (ADPKD).** This is usually diagnosed in adulthood.
- **Autosomal recessive PKD (ARPKD).** This can be diagnosed in the womb or shortly after a baby is born.

HOW COMMON IS POLYCYSTIC KIDNEY DISEASE?

Polycystic kidney disease is one of the most common genetic disorders. PKD affects about 500,000 people in the United States. ADPKD affects 1 in every 400–1,000 people in the world, and ARPKD affects 1 in 20,000 children.

WHO IS MORE LIKELY TO HAVE POLYCYSTIC KIDNEY DISEASE?

Polycystic kidney disease affects people of all ages, races, and ethnicities worldwide. The disorder occurs equally in women and men.

WHAT CAUSES POLYCYSTIC KIDNEY DISEASE?

A gene mutation, or defect, causes PKD. In most PKD cases, a child receives the gene mutation from a parent. In some PKD cases, the gene mutation develops on its own, without either parent carrying a copy of the mutated gene. This type of mutation is called "spontaneous."

WHAT ARE THE SIGNS AND SYMPTOMS OF POLYCYSTIC KIDNEY DISEASE?

The signs and symptoms of ADPKD, such as pain, HBP, and kidney failure, are also PKD complications. In many cases, ADPKD does not cause signs or symptoms until your kidney cysts are a half inch or larger.

Early signs of ARPKD in the womb are larger-than-normal kidneys and a smaller-than-average size baby, a condition called "growth failure." The early signs of ARPKD are also complications. However, some people with ARPKD do not develop signs or symptoms until later in childhood or even adulthood.

CAN I PREVENT POLYCYSTIC KIDNEY DISEASE?

Researchers have not yet found a way to prevent PKD. However, you may be able to slow PKD problems caused by HBP, such as kidney damage. Aim for a blood pressure goal of less than 120/80. Work with a health-care team to help manage your or your child's PKD. The health-care team will probably include a general practitioner and a nephrologist, a health-care provider specializing in kidney health.

WHAT CAN I DO TO SLOW DOWN POLYCYSTIC KIDNEY DISEASE?

The sooner you know you or your child has PKD, the sooner you can keep the condition from getting worse. Getting tested if you or your child are at risk for PKD can help you take early action.

You can also take steps to help delay or prevent kidney failure. Healthy lifestyle practices such as being active, reducing stress, and quitting smoking can help.

Make Lifestyle Changes

- **Be active.** Be active for 30 minutes or more on most days. Regular physical activity can help you reduce stress, manage your weight, and control your blood pressure. If you are not active now, ask your health-care provider about how much and what type of physical activity is right for you. If you play contact sports, such as football or hockey, a health-care provider should do a magnetic resonance imaging (MRI) test to see whether these sports are safe for you. Trauma to your body, especially to your back and sides, may cause kidney cysts to burst.
- **Lose weight.** Being overweight makes your kidneys work harder. Losing weight helps protect your kidneys.

- **Aim for seven to eight hours of sleep each night**. Getting enough sleep is important to your overall physical and mental health and can help you manage your blood pressure and blood glucose, or blood sugar.
- **Reduce stress.** Long-term stress can raise your blood pressure and even lead to depression. Some of the steps you take to manage your PKD are also healthy ways to cope with stress. For example, getting enough physical activity and sleep helps reduce stress.
- **Quit smoking.** Cigarette smoking can raise your blood pressure, making your kidney damage worse. Quitting smoking may help you meet your blood pressure goals, which is good for your kidneys and can lower your chances of having a heart attack or stroke. Quitting smoking is even more important for people with PKD who have aneurysms. An aneurysm is a bulge in the wall of a blood vessel.

Change What You Eat and Drink

You may need to change what you eat and drink to help control your blood pressure and protect your kidneys. People with any kind of kidney disease, including PKD, should talk with a dietitian about which foods and drinks to include in their healthy eating plan and which may be harmful. Staying hydrated by drinking the right amount of fluid may help slow PKD's progress toward kidney failure.

Take Blood Pressure Medicines

If lifestyle and diet changes do not help control your blood pressure, a health-care provider may prescribe one or more blood pressure medicines. Two types of blood pressure medicines, angiotensin-converting enzyme (ACE) inhibitors and angiotensin receptor blockers (ARBs), may slow kidney disease and delay kidney failure. The names of these medicines end in –pril or –sartan.[1]

[1] "Polycystic Kidney Disease," National Institute of Diabetes and Digestive and Kidney Diseases (NIDDK), January 2017. Available online. URL: www.niddk.nih.gov/health-information/kidney-disease/polycystic-kidney-disease/all-content. Accessed October 19, 2024.

Section 12.2 | Bartter Syndrome

WHAT IS BARTTER SYNDROME?

Bartter syndrome is a group of very similar kidney disorders that cause an imbalance of potassium, sodium, chloride, and related molecules in the body. In some cases, Bartter syndrome becomes apparent before birth. The disorder can cause polyhydramnios, which is an increased volume of fluid surrounding the fetus (amniotic fluid). Polyhydramnios increases the risk of premature birth. Beginning in infancy, babies with Bartter syndrome often fail to grow and gain weight at the expected rate (failure to thrive). They lose excess amounts of salt (sodium chloride) in their urine, which leads to dehydration, constipation, and increased urine production (polyuria). In addition, large amounts of calcium are lost through the urine (hypercalciuria), which can cause weakening of the bones (osteopenia). Some calcium is deposited in the kidneys as they concentrate urine, leading to hardening of the kidney tissue (nephrocalcinosis). Bartter syndrome is also characterized by low levels of potassium in the blood (hypokalemia), which can result in muscle weakness, cramping, and fatigue. Rarely, affected children develop hearing loss caused by abnormalities in the inner ear (sensorineural deafness). One form begins before birth (antenatal) and is often more severe. The other form, often called the "classical form," begins in early childhood and tends to be less severe.

WHEN DO SYMPTOMS OF BARTTER SYNDROME BEGIN?

Symptoms of this disease may start to appear at a variety of ages. The age symptoms may begin to appear differs between diseases. Symptoms may begin in a single age range, or during several age ranges. The symptoms of some diseases may begin at any age. Knowing when symptoms may have appeared can help medical providers find the correct diagnosis.

WHAT CAUSES BARTTER SYNDROME?

Bartter syndrome is caused by genetic mutations, also known as "pathogenic variants." Genetic mutations can be hereditary when parents pass them down to their children, or they may occur randomly when cells are dividing. Genetic mutations may also result from contracted viruses, environmental factors, such as UV radiation from sunlight exposure, or a combination of any of these.

CAN BARTTER SYNDROME BE PASSED DOWN FROM PARENT TO CHILD?

Yes. It is possible for a biological parent to pass down genetic mutations that cause or increase the chances of getting this disease to their child. This is known as "inheritance." Knowing whether other family members have previously had this disease, also known as "family health history," can be very important information for your medical team.

Autosomal Dominant

Autosomal means the gene involved is located on one of the numbered chromosomes. Dominant means that a child only needs to inherit one copy of the mutated gene from either biological parent to be affected by the disease. People affected by an autosomal dominant disease have a 50 percent chance of passing on the mutated gene to their biological child.

Autosomal Recessive

Autosomal means the gene involved is located on one of the numbered chromosomes. Recessive means that a child must inherit two copies of the mutated gene, one from each biological parent, to be affected by the disease. A carrier is a person who only has one copy of the genetic mutation. A carrier usually does not show any symptoms of the disease. If both biological parents are carriers, there is a 25 percent chance their child inherits both copies of the mutated gene and is affected by the disease. Additionally, there is a 50 percent chance their child inherits only one copy of the mutated gene and is a carrier.

X-Linked

X-linked inheritance means the genetic mutation is located on the X chromosome, one of the sex chromosomes. The male sex chromosome pair consists of one X and one Y chromosome (XY). The female sex chromosome pair consists of two X chromosomes

(XX). Because males have just one X chromosome, it takes only one copy of the mutated gene to cause the disease. Females that have one copy of the mutated gene may have symptoms similar to those experienced by affected males but usually have less severe symptoms or no symptoms at all. Female parents with one X-linked mutated gene have a 50 percent chance of passing on the mutation to each of their biological children. Male parents with an X-linked mutated gene will pass on the mutation to all their female children but cannot pass the mutation on to their male children.

HOW CAN PATIENT ORGANIZATIONS HELP?

Patient organizations can help patients and families connect. They build public awareness of the disease and are a driving force behind research to improve patients' lives. They may offer online and in-person resources to help people live well with their disease. Many collaborate with medical experts and researchers.

Services of patient organizations differ but may include:

- ways to connect to others and share personal stories
- easy-to-read information
- up-to-date treatment and research information
- patient registries
- lists of specialists or specialty centers
- financial aid and travel resources[1]

Section 12.3 | **Ectopic Kidney**

WHAT IS AN ECTOPIC KIDNEY?

An ectopic kidney is a kidney located below, above, or on the opposite side of the kidney's normal position in the urinary tract. The two kidneys are usually located near the middle of your back, just below your rib cage, on either side of your spine.

[1] Genetic and Rare Diseases Information Center (GARD), "Bartter Syndrome," National Center for Advancing Translational Sciences (NCATS), August 2024. Available online. URL: https://rarediseases.info.nih.gov/diseases/5893/bartter-syndrome. Accessed October 19, 2024.

An ectopic kidney usually does not cause any symptoms or health problems, and many people never find out that they have the condition. If an ectopic kidney is discovered, it is usually found during a fetal ultrasound—an imaging test that uses sound waves to create a picture of how a baby is developing in the womb—or during medical tests done to check for a urinary tract infection or to find the cause of abdominal pain. Rarely does a person have two ectopic kidneys.

In the womb, a fetus's kidneys first develop as small buds in the lower abdomen inside the pelvis. During the first eight weeks of growth, the fetus's kidneys slowly move from the pelvis to their normal position in the back near the rib cage. When an ectopic kidney occurs during growth, the kidney:

- stays in the pelvis near the bladder
- stops moving up too early and stays in the lower abdomen
- moves too high up in the abdomen
- crosses over the center of the body and often grows into or joins the other kidney, with both kidneys on the same side of the body

DOES AN ECTOPIC KIDNEY HAVE ANOTHER NAME?

When the kidney stays in the pelvis, it is called a "pelvic kidney." If the kidney crosses to the other side of the body, it is called "crossed renal ectopia" (see Figures 12.2 and 12.3).

WHAT CAUSES AN ECTOPIC KIDNEY?

An ectopic kidney is a birth defect that happens while the fetus is developing. Researchers do not know exactly what causes most birth defects, including the ectopic kidney.

An ectopic kidney may result from:

- a poorly developed kidney bud
- a problem in the kidney tissue that directs the developing kidney where to move
- a genetic defect that causes a genetic disorder
- an illness, infection, or drug or chemical reaction during fetal growth

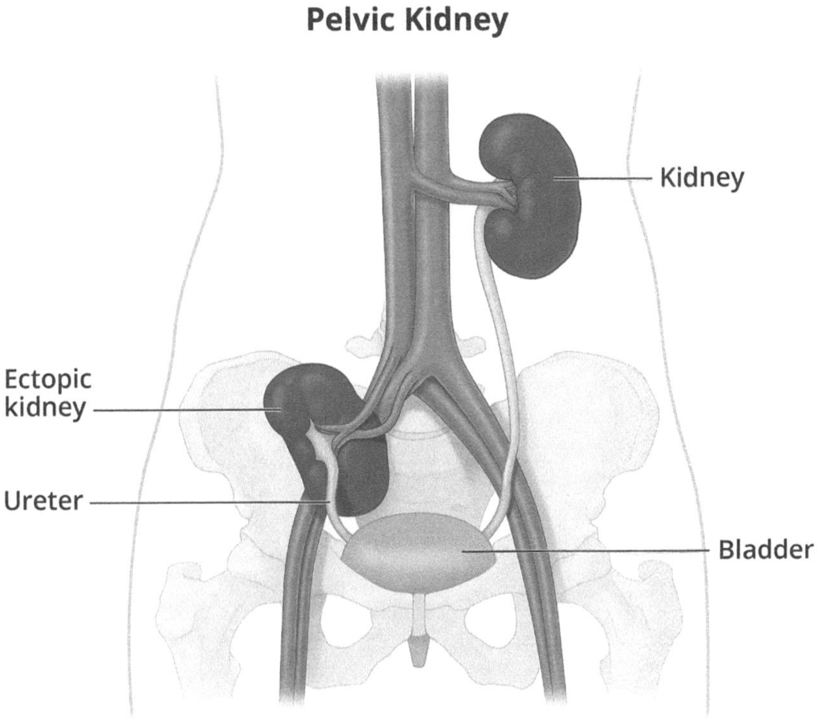

Figure 12.2. Pelvic Kidney

National Institute of Diabetes and Digestive and Kidney Diseases (NIDDK)

HOW COMMON IS AN ECTOPIC KIDNEY?

Most people who have an ectopic kidney do not have symptoms, so researchers do not know exactly how many people have one. Some studies suggest about 1 in 1,000 people has an ectopic kidney.

WHAT OTHER HEALTH PROBLEMS CAN AN ECTOPIC KIDNEY CAUSE?

An ectopic kidney usually does not cause health problems or complications and may work normally. Most people are born with two kidneys, so if your ectopic kidney does not work at all, your other kidney may be able to do the work both kidneys would have done.

In rare cases, a nonfunctioning ectopic kidney must be removed. As long as the other kidney is working well, there should be no problems living with one kidney, also called a "solitary kidney."

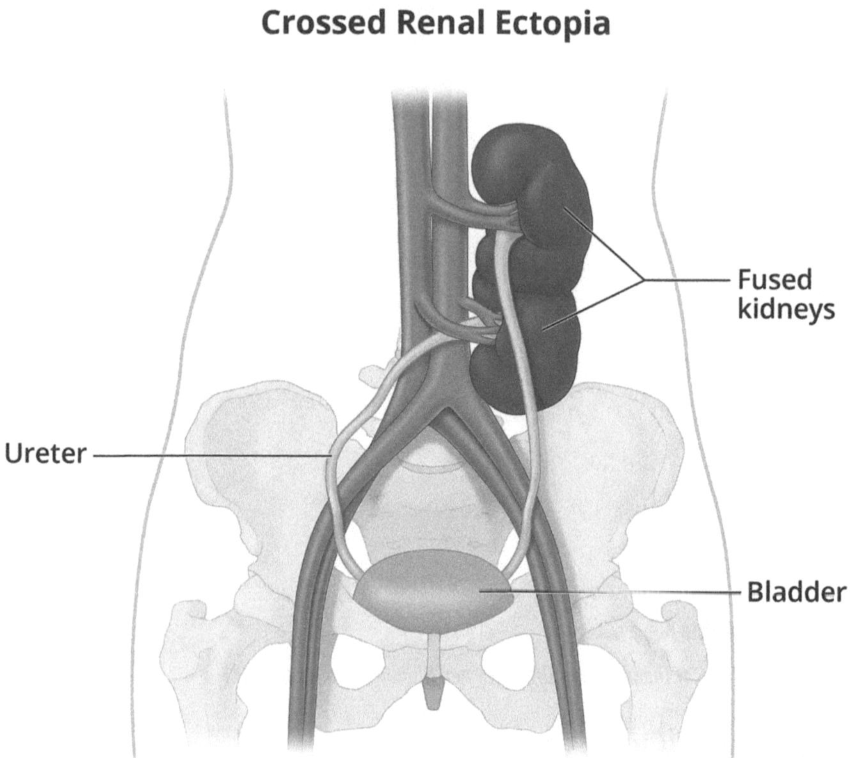

Figure 12.3. Crossed Renal Ectopia

National Institute of Diabetes and Digestive and Kidney Diseases (NIDDK)

People who have an ectopic kidney are more likely to have vesicoureteral reflux (VUR). VUR is a condition in which urine flows backward from the bladder to one or both ureters and sometimes to the kidneys. In some people, an ectopic kidney can block urine from correctly draining from the body or may be associated with VUR.

The abnormal placement of the ectopic kidney and potential problems with slow or blocked urine flow can be associated with other problems, including:

- **Urinary tract infection**. In a urinary tract with slow or blocked urine drainage or VUR, bacteria in the urine is not flushed out of the urinary tract as it normally would be, which may lead to a urinary tract infection.
- **Kidney stones**. Kidney stones, also called "urinary tract calculi," develop from minerals typically found in the urine, such as calcium and oxalate. When urine drainage is slower than normal, these minerals are more likely to build up and form kidney stones.
- **Trauma**. An ectopic kidney in your lower abdomen or pelvis or a fused ectopic kidney may be at greater risk for damage from certain kinds of injury or trauma. Talk with a health-care professional if you or your child has an ectopic kidney and wants to play contact sports or participate in other activities that may result in injury to the kidney. Talk with your health-care professional about treatment options if you have any of these health problems.

WHAT ARE THE SYMPTOMS OF AN ECTOPIC KIDNEY?

Most people with an ectopic kidney have no symptoms. If complications occur, however, symptoms may include:

- pain in your abdomen or back
- urinary frequency or urgency, or burning during urination
- fever
- hematuria, or blood in the urine
- lump or mass in the abdomen
- high blood pressure (HBP)

HOW DO HEALTH-CARE PROFESSIONALS DIAGNOSE AN ECTOPIC KIDNEY?

Many people who have an ectopic kidney do not discover it unless they have tests done for other reasons or the ectopic kidney was found during a prenatal ultrasound.

Health-care professionals may use urinary tract imaging tests and lab tests to determine whether you have an ectopic kidney and rule out other health problems. If your ectopic kidney is not causing symptoms or other health problems, you usually do not need further testing or treatment.

Imaging Tests

A specially trained technician performs imaging tests at an outpatient center or hospital, and a radiologist reviews the images. Health-care professionals use the following imaging tests to help diagnose and manage an ectopic kidney:

- Ultrasounds use sound waves to examine internal body structures, including the location of the kidneys.
- Voiding cystourethrograms use x-rays to show how urine flows through the bladder and urethra.
- Radionuclide scans, also called "nuclear scans," may show the location and size of an ectopic kidney and may show any blockages in the urinary system.
- Magnetic resonance imaging (MRI) can show the location, size, shape, and function of the kidneys.

Lab Tests

A health-care professional may do urine and blood tests to test your kidney function.

HOW DO HEALTH-CARE PROFESSIONALS TREAT AN ECTOPIC KIDNEY?

Your health-care professional may not need to treat your ectopic kidney if it is not causing symptoms or damage to your body or kidney. If tests show that you have a blockage or other potential complication in the urinary tract, your health-care professional may suggest further follow-up or surgery to correct the abnormality.

If you have VUR with symptoms, a health-care professional can evaluate and manage your VUR.[1]

[1] "Ectopic Kidney," National Institute of Diabetes and Digestive and Kidney Diseases (NIDDK), September 2019. Available online. URL: www.niddk.nih.gov/health-information/kidney-disease/children/ectopic-kidney. Accessed October 19, 2024.

Section 12.4 | Fabry Disease

WHAT IS FABRY DISEASE?

Fabry disease is a type of lysosomal storage disease. Lysosomes are round structures found in the cells of the body that are full of special proteins called "enzymes." Lysosomal enzymes help break down other proteins, carbohydrates, fats, and other substances. In Fabry disease, there is not enough of the enzyme alpha-galactosidase (alpha-GAL). Alpha-GAL helps break down a fatty acid called "globotriaosylceramide" or "GL-3." Without enough alpha-GAL, the lysosomes become filled with GL-3 and cannot function properly. Symptoms of Fabry disease may include episodes of pain, especially in the hands and feet, clusters of small, dark red spots on the skin called "angiokeratomas," a decreased ability to sweat (hypohidrosis), cloudiness of the front part of the eye (corneal opacity), and hearing loss. Internal organs, such as the kidneys, heart, or brain, may also be affected, leading to progressive kidney damage, heart attacks, and strokes. Milder forms of Fabry disease may appear later in life and affect only the heart or kidneys. Fabry disease is caused by certain changes (pathogenic variants, also called "genetic changes") in the GLA gene. Since the GLA gene is located on the X chromosome, Fabry disease is inherited in an X-linked manner. Although an enzyme assay test measuring the activity of alpha-GAL can diagnose Fabry disease in males, diagnosis is usually made by genetic testing in both males and females.

SYMPTOMS

The types of symptoms experienced and their intensity may vary among people with this disease. Your experience may be different from others. Consult your health-care team for more information.

WHAT CAUSES THIS DISEASE?

Genetic Mutations

Fabry disease is caused by genetic mutations, also known as "pathogenic variants." Genetic mutations can be hereditary when parents pass them down to their children, or they may occur randomly when cells are dividing. Genetic mutations may also result from contracted viruses, environmental factors, such as ultraviolet (UV) radiation from sunlight exposure, or a combination of any of these.

Disruption in Metabolism

Fabry disease is caused by a disruption in a person's metabolism. Metabolism is the series of chemical reactions in our body that turns the food we eat into energy and removes toxins. Hormones and specific proteins, called "enzymes," help make the right chemical reactions happen in the right order. However, genetic changes can prevent hormones or enzymes from working properly, which can lead to a disruption in metabolism, such as energy not being created for the body or toxins not being removed from the body.

Impaired Lysosomal Function

This disease is caused by an impairment, or issue, in lysosomal function. Lysosomes are located inside cells and contain digestive enzymes that help break down fats, sugars, and other substances to create energy for the body. Genetic mutations can affect lysosomes, such as having a missing or non-functioning digestive enzyme. This can prevent cells from properly breaking down toxins or moving them out of the cell. If toxins build up, the cell may become damaged or die. Depending on their location in the body, these damaged or dead cells may affect different organs and body systems.

CAN THIS DISEASE BE PASSED DOWN FROM PARENT TO CHILD?

Yes. It is possible for a biological parent to pass down genetic mutations that cause or increase the chances of getting this disease to their child. This is known as "inheritance." Knowing whether other family members have previously had this disease, also known as "family health history," can be very important information for your medical team.

X-Linked

X-linked inheritance means the genetic mutation is located on the X chromosome, one of the sex chromosomes. The male sex chromosome pair consists of one X and one Y chromosome (XY). The female sex chromosome pair consists of two X chromosomes (XX). Because males have just one X chromosome, it takes only one copy of the mutated gene to cause the disease. Females that have one copy of the mutated gene may have symptoms similar to those experienced by affected males, but usually have less severe symptoms or no symptoms at all. Female parents with one X-linked mutated gene have a 50 percent chance of passing on the mutation to each of their biological children. Male parents with an X-linked mutated gene will pass on the mutation to all their female children but cannot pass the mutation on to their male children.

HOW CAN PATIENT ORGANIZATIONS HELP?

Patient organizations can help patients and families connect. They build public awareness of the disease and are a driving force behind research to improve patients' lives. They may offer online and in-person resources to help people live well with their disease. Many collaborate with medical experts and researchers.

Services of patient organizations differ but may include:

- ways to connect to others and share personal stories
- easy-to-read information
- up-to-date treatment and research information
- patient registries
- lists of specialists or specialty centers
- financial aid and travel resources[1]

[1] Genetic and Rare Diseases Information Center (GARD), "Fabry Disease," National Center for Advancing Translational Sciences (NCATS), September 2024. Available online. URL: https://rarediseases.info.nih.gov/diseases/6400/fabry-disease. Accessed October 19, 2024.

Section 12.5 | **Medullary Sponge Kidney**

WHAT IS MEDULLARY SPONGE KIDNEY?

Medullary sponge kidney, also known as "Cacchi-Ricci disease," is a birth defect where changes occur in the tubules, or tiny tubes, inside a fetus's kidneys.

In a normal kidney, urine flows through these tubules as the kidney is being formed during a fetus's growth. In medullary sponge kidney, tiny, fluid-filled sacs called "cysts" form in the tubules within the medulla—the inner part of the kidney—creating a sponge-like appearance. The cysts keep urine from flowing freely through the tubules (see Figure 12.4).

Symptoms of medullary sponge kidney do not usually appear until the teenage years or the 20s. Medullary sponge kidney can affect one or both kidneys.

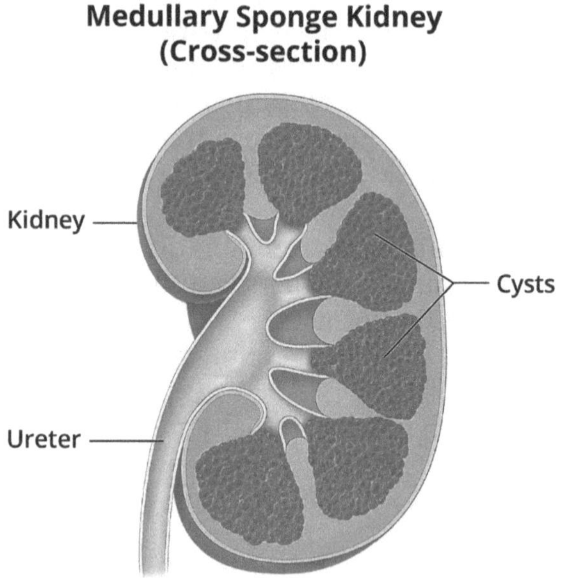

Figure 12.4. Medullary Sponge Kidney

National Institute of Diabetes and Digestive and Kidney Diseases (NIDDK)

WHAT ARE THE COMPLICATIONS OF MEDULLARY SPONGE KIDNEY?

Complications of medullary sponge kidney include:

- hematuria, or blood in the urine
- kidney stones
- urinary tract infections (UTIs)

Medullary sponge kidney rarely leads to more serious problems, such as chronic kidney disease or kidney failure.

WHAT CAUSES MEDULLARY SPONGE KIDNEY?

Scientists do not fully understand the cause of the medullary sponge kidney or why cysts form in the tubules during fetal development. Even though the medullary sponge kidney is present at birth, most cases do not appear to be inherited.

HOW COMMON IS MEDULLARY SPONGE KIDNEY?

Medullary sponge kidney affects about 1 person per 5,000 people in the United States. Researchers have reported that 12–20 percent of people who develop calcium-based kidney stones have medullary sponge kidney.

WHO IS MORE LIKELY TO DEVELOP MEDULLARY SPONGE KIDNEY?

The medullary sponge kidney affects all races and geographic regions. Among people who are more likely to develop calcium-based kidney stones, women are more likely than men to have medullary sponge kidney.

WHAT ARE THE SIGNS AND SYMPTOMS OF MEDULLARY SPONGE KIDNEY?

Many people with the medullary sponge kidney have no symptoms. The first sign that a person has a medullary sponge kidney is usually a UTI or a kidney stone. UTIs and kidney stones share many of the same signs and symptoms:

- burning or painful urination
- pain in the back, lower abdomen, or groin
- cloudy, dark, or bloody urine
- foul-smelling urine
- fever and chills
- vomiting

People who experience these symptoms should see or call a health-care provider as soon as possible.

HOW IS MEDULLARY SPONGE KIDNEY DIAGNOSED?

A health-care provider diagnoses medullary sponge kidney based on:

- a medical and family history
- a physical exam
- imaging studies

Medical and Family History

Taking a medical and family history can help diagnose medullary sponge kidney. A health-care provider will suspect medullary sponge kidney when a person has repeated UTIs or kidney stones.

Physical Exam

A patient with a medullary sponge kidney usually has no physical signs except for blood in the urine. Health-care providers usually confirm a diagnosis of medullary sponge kidney with imaging studies.

Imaging Studies

Imaging is the medical term for tests that use different methods to see bones, tissues, and organs inside the body. Health-care providers commonly choose one or more of three imaging techniques to diagnose medullary sponge kidney:

- intravenous pyelogram
- computerized tomography (CT) scan
- ultrasound

A radiologist—a doctor who specializes in medical imaging—interprets the images from these studies, and patients do not need anesthesia.

INTRAVENOUS PYELOGRAM

In an intravenous pyelogram, a health-care provider injects a special dye, called "contrast medium," into a vein in the patient's arm. The contrast medium travels through the body to the kidneys. The kidneys excrete the contrast medium into the urine, which makes the urine visible on an x-ray. An x-ray technician performs this procedure at a health-care provider's office, an outpatient center, or a hospital. An intravenous pyelogram can show any blockage in the urinary tract, and the cysts show up as clusters of light.

COMPUTERIZED TOMOGRAPHY SCANS

Computerized tomography scans use a combination of x-rays and computer technology to create images. For a CT scan, a health-care provider may give the patient a solution to drink and an injection of contrast medium. CT scans require the patient to lie on a table that slides into a tunnel-shaped device where the x-rays are taken. An x-ray technician performs the procedure in an outpatient center or a hospital. CT scans can show expanded or stretched tubules.

ULTRASOUND

Ultrasound uses a device called a "transducer" that bounces safe, painless sound waves off organs to create an image of their structure. A specially trained technician performs the procedure in a health-care provider's office, an outpatient center, or a hospital. Ultrasound can show kidney stones and calcium deposits within the kidney.

HOW IS MEDULLARY SPONGE KIDNEY TREATED?

Scientists have not discovered a way to reverse the medullary sponge kidney. Once a health-care provider is sure a person has medullary sponge kidney, treatment focuses on:

- curing an existing UTI
- removing any kidney stones

Curing an Existing Urinary Tract Infection

To treat a UTI, the health-care provider may prescribe a medication called an "antibiotic" that kills bacteria. The choice of medication and length of treatment depend on the person's medical history and the type of bacteria causing the infection.

Removing Kidney Stones

Treatment for kidney stones usually depends on their size and composition, as well as whether they are causing pain or obstructing the urinary tract. Kidney stones may be treated by a general practitioner or by a urologist—a doctor who specializes in the urinary tract.

Small stones usually pass through the urinary tract without treatment. Still, the person may need pain medication and should drink lots of liquids to help move the stone along. Pain control may consist of oral or intravenous (IV) medication, depending on the duration and severity of the pain. People may need IV fluids if they become dehydrated from vomiting or an inability to drink.

A person with a larger stone, or one that blocks urine flow and causes great pain, may need more urgent treatment, such as:

- **Shock wave lithotripsy**. A machine called a "lithotripter" breaks up the kidney stone into smaller pieces so it can pass more easily through the urinary tract. The patient may need local or general anesthesia.
- **Ureteroscopy**. A ureteroscope—a long, tube-like instrument with an eyepiece—is used to find and retrieve the stone with a small basket or to break the stone up with laser energy. Local or general anesthesia may be required.
- **Percutaneous nephrolithotomy**. In this procedure, a wire-thin viewing instrument called a "nephroscope" is used to locate and remove the stones. During the procedure, which requires general anesthesia, a tube is inserted directly into the kidney through a small incision in the patient's back.

CAN MEDULLARY SPONGE KIDNEY BE PREVENTED?

Scientists have not yet found a way to prevent medullary sponge kidney. However, health-care providers can recommend medications and dietary changes to prevent future UTIs and kidney stones.

Medications to Prevent Future Urinary Tract Infections and Kidney Stones

Health-care providers may prescribe certain medications to prevent UTIs and kidney stones:

- A person with a medullary sponge kidney may need to continue taking a low-dose antibiotic to prevent recurrent infections.
- Medications that reduce calcium in the urine, such as potassium citrate and thiazide, may help prevent kidney stones.

Eating, Diet, and Nutrition

The following changes in diet may help prevent UTIs and kidney stone formation:

- **Drinking plenty of water and other liquids can help flush bacteria from the urinary tract and dilute urine so kidney stones cannot form.** A person should drink enough liquid to produce about 2–2.5 quarts of urine every day.
- **Reducing sodium intake, mostly from salt, may help prevent kidney stones.** Diets high in sodium can increase the excretion of calcium into the urine and thus increase the chance of calcium-containing kidney stones forming.
- **Foods rich in animal proteins such as meat, eggs, and fish can increase the chance of uric acid stones and calcium stones forming.** People who form stones should limit their meat consumption to 6–8 ounces a day.
- **People who are more likely to develop calcium oxalate stones should include 1,000 milligrams of calcium in their diet every day.** Adults older than 50 years should consume 1,200 milligrams of calcium

daily. Calcium in the digestive tract binds to oxalate from food and keeps it from entering the blood and the urinary tract, where it can form stones.

People with the medullary sponge kidney should talk with their health-care provider or a dietitian before making any dietary changes. A dietitian can help a person plan healthy meals.[1]

Section 12.6 | **Primary Hyperoxaluria**

WHAT IS PRIMARY HYPEROXALURIA?

Primary hyperoxaluria is a rare condition characterized by recurrent kidney and bladder stones. The condition often results in end-stage renal disease (ESRD), which is a life-threatening condition that prevents the kidneys from filtering fluids and waste products from the body effectively.

Primary hyperoxaluria results from the overproduction of a substance called "oxalate." Oxalate is filtered through the kidneys and excreted as a waste product in urine, leading to abnormally high levels of this substance in urine (hyperoxaluria). During its excretion, oxalate can combine with calcium to form calcium oxalate, a hard compound that is the main component of kidney and bladder stones. Deposits of calcium oxalate can damage the kidneys and other organs and lead to blood in the urine (hematuria), urinary tract infections, kidney damage, ESRD, and injury to other organs. Over time, kidney function decreases such that the kidneys can no longer excrete as much oxalate as they receive. As a result, oxalate levels in the blood rise, and the substance gets deposited in tissues throughout the body (systemic oxalosis), particularly in bones and the walls of blood vessels. Oxalosis in bones can cause fractures.

[1] "Medullary Sponge Kidney," National Institute of Diabetes and Digestive and Kidney Diseases (NIDDK), August 2015. Available online. URL: www.niddk.nih.gov/health-information/kidney-disease/children/medullary-sponge-kidney. Accessed October 22, 2024.

TYPES OF PRIMARY HYPEROXALURIA

There are three types of primary hyperoxaluria that differ in their severity and genetic cause. In primary hyperoxaluria type 1, kidney stones typically begin to appear anytime from childhood to early adulthood, and ESRD can develop at any age. Primary hyperoxaluria type 2 is similar to type 1, but ESRD develops later in life. In primary hyperoxaluria type 3, affected individuals often develop kidney stones in early childhood, but few cases of this type have been described, so additional signs and symptoms of this type are unclear.[1]

Primary Hyperoxaluria Type 1

Primary hyperoxaluria type 1 (PH1) is a rare disorder that mainly affects the kidneys. It results from the buildup of a substance called "oxalate," which normally is filtered through the kidneys and excreted in the urine. In people with PH1, the accumulated oxalate is deposited in the kidneys and urinary tract. It combines with calcium, forming the main component of kidney and bladder stones (calcium oxalate). Signs and symptoms of PH1 vary in severity and may begin any time from infancy to early adulthood. Symptoms may include recurrent kidney stones, blood in the urine, and urinary tract infections. PH1 is due to genetic changes in a gene called "*AGXT*." Inheritance is autosomal recessive.[2]

Primary Hyperoxaluria Type 2

Primary hyperoxaluria type 2 is a rare condition characterized by the overproduction of a substance called "oxalate" (also called "oxalic acid"). In the kidneys, the excess oxalate combines with calcium to form calcium oxalate, a hard compound that is the main component of kidney stones. Deposits of calcium oxalate can lead to kidney damage, kidney failure, and injury to other organs. Primary hyperoxaluria type 2 is caused by the shortage

---

[1] MedlinePlus, "Primary Hyperoxaluria," National Institutes of Health (NIH), December 1, 2015. Available online. URL: https://medlineplus.gov/genetics/condition/primary-hyperoxaluria. Accessed October 16, 2024.
[2] Genetic and Rare Diseases Information Center (GARD), "Primary Hyperoxaluria Type 1," National Center for Advancing Translational Sciences (NCATS), August 2024. Available online. URL: https://rarediseases.info.nih.gov/diseases/2835/primary-hyperoxaluria-type-1. Accessed October 16, 2024.

(deficiency) of an enzyme called "glyoxylate reductase/hydroxypyruvate reductase" (*GRHPR*) that normally prevents the buildup of oxalate. This enzyme shortage is caused by genetic changes in the *GRHPR* gene. Primary hyperoxaluria type 2 is inherited in an autosomal recessive pattern.[3]

FREQUENCY OF PRIMARY HYPEROXALURIA

Primary hyperoxaluria is estimated to affect 1 in 58,000 people worldwide. Type 1 is the most common form, accounting for approximately 80 percent of cases. Types 2 and 3 each account for about 10 percent of cases.

CAUSES OF PRIMARY HYPEROXALURIA

Mutations in the *AGXT*, *GRHPR*, and *HOGA1* genes cause primary hyperoxaluria types 1, 2, and 3, respectively. These genes provide instructions for making enzymes involved in the breakdown and processing of protein building blocks (amino acids) and other compounds. The enzyme produced from the *HOGA1* gene is involved in the breakdown of an amino acid, which results in the formation of a compound called "glyoxylate." The enzymes produced from the *AGXT* and *GRHPR* genes further break down this compound.

Mutations in the *AGXT*, *GRHPR*, or *HOGA1* genes lead to a decrease in the production or activity of the respective proteins, which prevents the normal breakdown of glyoxylate. *AGXT* and *GRHPR* gene mutations result in an accumulation of glyoxylate, which is then converted to oxalate for removal from the body as a waste product. *HOGA1* gene mutations also result in excess oxalate, although researchers are unsure how this occurs. Oxalate that is not excreted from the body combines with calcium to form calcium oxalate deposits, which can damage the kidneys and other organs.

[3] Genetic and Rare Diseases Information Center (GARD), "Primary Hyperoxaluria Type 2," National Center for Advancing Translational Sciences (NCATS), August 2024. Available online. URL: https://rarediseases.info.nih.gov/diseases/2836/primary-hyperoxaluria-type-2. Accessed October 16, 2024.

INHERITANCE OF PRIMARY HYPEROXALURIA

This condition is inherited in an autosomal recessive pattern, which means both copies of the gene in each cell have mutations. The parents of an individual with an autosomal recessive condition each carry one copy of the mutated gene, but they typically do not show signs and symptoms of the condition.[4]

Section 12.7 | **Solitary Kidney**

WHAT IS A SOLITARY KIDNEY?

If only one kidney is present, that kidney is called a "solitary kidney" (see Figure 12.5). This condition is different from having a solitary functioning kidney, in which two kidneys are present, but only one is functioning.

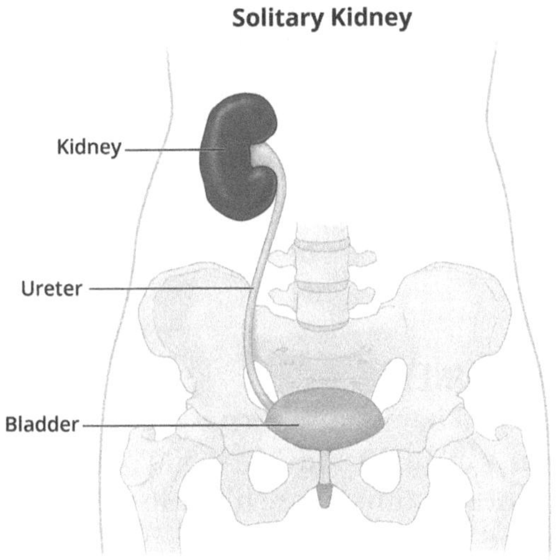

Figure 12.5. Solitary Kidney

National Institute of Diabetes and Digestive and Kidney Diseases (NIDDK)

[4] See footnote [1].

WHAT CAUSES A SOLITARY KIDNEY?

The three main causes of a solitary kidney are:

- **Birth defects.** Some people are born with only one kidney because the other kidney never developed—a condition known as "renal agenesis" or "kidney agenesis." A solitary kidney is sometimes diagnosed before birth by a routine prenatal ultrasound; sometimes, it is diagnosed later in life after an x-ray, an ultrasound, or surgery for an unrelated clinical condition.
- **Some people are born with one normal kidney and another abnormal, nonfunctioning kidney that may eventually shrink, making it no longer visible on x-ray or ultrasound.** This condition is known as "kidney dysplasia" (see Figure 12.6).
- **Surgical removal of a kidney.** Some people must have a kidney removed to treat kidney cancer or another disease or injury. This surgery is known as a "nephrectomy." When a kidney is removed surgically, the ureter is also removed.
- **Kidney donation.** A growing number of people are donating a kidney to be transplanted into a family member or friend whose kidneys have failed. Many people even donate a kidney to a stranger in need.

HOW COMMON IS A SOLITARY KIDNEY?

Globally, an estimated 1 in 2,000 babies are born each year with kidney agenesis, and between 1 in 1,000 and 1 in 4,300 babies are born with kidney dysplasia. These estimates are likely low because some babies are never diagnosed with these conditions, particularly in countries where pregnant women do not routinely undergo prenatal ultrasounds.

Between 2008 and 2017, more than 58,000 Americans donated a kidney as living donors, and more than 255,000 people had a kidney surgically removed to treat cancer, leaving them with solitary kidneys.

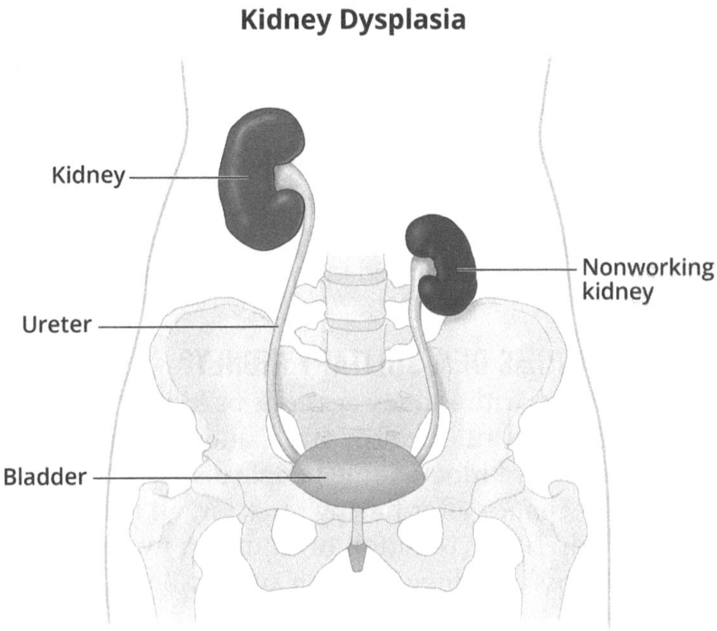

Figure 12.6. Kidney Dysplasia

National Institute of Diabetes and Digestive and Kidney Diseases (NIDDK)

WHO IS MORE LIKELY TO HAVE A SOLITARY KIDNEY?

Men are more likely than women to be born with a solitary kidney and to receive donated kidneys. Women, however, are more likely than men to be living kidney donors.

WHAT ARE THE COMPLICATIONS OF A SOLITARY KIDNEY?

Complications from a solitary kidney are rare but may include:

- increased protein in the urine, known as "albuminuria"
- a lower-than-normal glomerular filtration rate (GFR), which measures how quickly the kidneys filter wastes and extra fluid from the blood—while less common, this complication can sometimes lead to kidney failure

- high blood pressure (HBP)
- high blood pressure during pregnancy—this complication less commonly results in organ damage in the mother or child, a condition known as "preeclampsia"

People with kidney agenesis or kidney dysplasia can be at an increased risk for developing kidney disease. For example, if the solitary kidney functioned normally during childhood, there is still an increased risk of having decreased kidney function as an adult.

WHAT ARE THE SYMPTOMS OF A SOLITARY KIDNEY?

In general, people born with kidney agenesis or kidney dysplasia show no symptoms, lead full healthy lives, and may never discover they have a solitary kidney. Some people discover they have a solitary kidney by chance after having an x-ray, an ultrasound, or surgery for an unrelated condition or injury. A minority may develop progressive loss of kidney function and can develop symptoms associated with chronic kidney disease.

A small percentage of babies born with kidney agenesis have other birth defects, such as an absent anus, an absent or smaller-than-normal bladder, an absent or smaller-than-normal uterus, a smaller-than-normal lung, club feet, or a hole in the heart wall separating the two lower heart chambers.

HOW DO HEALTH-CARE PROFESSIONALS DIAGNOSE A SOLITARY KIDNEY?

During pregnancy, a health-care professional can diagnose kidney agenesis and kidney dysplasia while conducting a prenatal ultrasound. Ultrasound uses a device called a "transducer" that bounces safe, painless sound waves off the fetus's organs to create an image of their structure. Ultrasounds during pregnancy are part of routine prenatal testing.

If a fetus is diagnosed with kidney agenesis or kidney dysplasia, health-care professionals may recommend additional ultrasounds before and after the birth to find out how the solitary kidney functions over time and to check for other health problems.

In adults, health-care professionals may diagnose a solitary kidney during an x-ray, ultrasound, or surgery for another condition or injury.

HOW DO HEALTH-CARE PROFESSIONALS TREAT A SOLITARY KIDNEY?

If a solitary kidney is present, the health-care professional will take the following actions:

- Monitor kidney function by conducting urine and, sometimes, blood tests.
- Monitor and control blood pressure.

Testing Blood and Urine

A health-care professional uses two types of tests to monitor kidney function:

- a blood test that checks how well the kidneys are filtering blood, called the "glomerular filtration rate" (GFR)
- a urine test to check for albumin, a protein that can pass into the urine when the kidneys are damaged

In some cases, additional tests may be performed to measure kidney function.

Monitoring and Controlling Blood Pressure

High blood pressure can damage blood vessels in the solitary kidney. If the kidneys' blood vessels are damaged, they may no longer work properly. When this happens, the kidney is unable to remove all wastes and extra fluid from the body. Extra fluid in the blood vessels can raise blood pressure even more, creating a dangerous cycle and causing further damage leading to kidney failure.

If a diagnosis of high blood pressure is made, the health-care professional may prescribe one or more blood pressure-lowering medicines. Medicines that lower blood pressure can also significantly slow the progression of kidney disease.

Two types of blood pressure-lowering medicines, angiotensin-converting enzyme (ACE) inhibitors and angiotensin receptor blockers (ARBs), may be effective in slowing kidney disease progression while also lowering blood pressure. A health-care professional may also prescribe a diuretic.

CAN INJURY TO A SOLITARY KIDNEY BE PREVENTED?

Health-care professionals should be informed if a solitary kidney is present to prevent injury from medications or medical procedures. Certain sports may be more likely to injure the kidney. This risk is particularly concerning for children, as they are more likely to engage in sports. Consultation with a health-care professional regarding specific sports and strategies to reduce the risk of injury is advisable. Loss of the remaining functioning kidney will result in the need for dialysis or a kidney transplant.

HOW DO EATING, DIET, AND NUTRITION AFFECT A SOLITARY KIDNEY?

If a solitary kidney is present, there is no need for a special diet. However, maintaining kidney health can be supported by staying well-hydrated, minimizing salt intake, and avoiding excessive weight gain. If reduced kidney function is present, dietary changes may be necessary to slow the progression of kidney disease. Collaboration with a health-care professional or registered dietitian is recommended to develop a meal plan that includes enjoyable foods while promoting kidney health.[1]

Section 12.8 | **Nephrogenic Diabetes Insipidus**

WHAT IS NEPHROGENIC DIABETES INSIPIDUS?

Nephrogenic diabetes insipidus is a disorder in which a defect in the small tubes (tubules) in the kidneys causes a person to

[1] "Solitary or Single-Functioning Kidney," National Institute of Diabetes and Digestive and Kidney Diseases (NIDDK), October 2020. Available online. URL: www.niddk.nih.gov/health-information/kidney-disease/solitary-kidney. Accessed October 22, 2024.

produce a large amount of urine. This condition occurs when the kidney tubules, which allow water to be removed from the body or reabsorbed, do not respond to a chemical in the body called "antidiuretic hormone" (ADH) or "vasopressin." ADH normally tells the kidneys to make the urine more concentrated. As a result of the defect, the kidneys release an excessive amount of water into the urine, producing a large quantity of very dilute urine. The most common symptoms are frequent urination (polyuria), especially during nighttime (nocturia), and excessive thirst (polydipsia). Nephrogenic diabetes insipidus can be either acquired or hereditary. The acquired form is brought on by certain drugs and chronic diseases and can occur at any time during life. About 90 percent of all cases of hereditary nephrogenic diabetes insipidus result from genetic changes in the *AVPR2* gene, and about 10 percent of cases are caused by genetic changes in the *AQP2* gene.

WHEN DO SYMPTOMS OF NEPHROGENIC DIABETES INSIPIDUS BEGIN?

Symptoms of this disease may start to appear in newborns and infants. The age at which symptoms may begin to appear differs between diseases. Symptoms may begin in a single age range or during several age ranges. The symptoms of some diseases may begin at any age. Knowing when symptoms may have appeared can help medical providers find the correct diagnosis.

WHAT CAUSES THIS DISEASE?

Genetic Mutations

Nephrogenic diabetes insipidus is caused by genetic mutations, also known as "pathogenic variants." Genetic mutations can be hereditary when parents pass them down to their children, or they may occur randomly when cells are dividing. Genetic mutations may also result from contracted viruses, environmental factors, such as UV radiation from sunlight exposure, or a combination of any of these.

Nephrogenic diabetes insipidus is caused by genetic mutations in the following known gene(s):

- *AQP2*
- *AVPR2*

CAN THIS DISEASE BE PASSED DOWN FROM PARENT TO CHILD?

Yes. It is possible for a biological parent to pass down genetic mutations that cause or increase the chances of getting this disease to their child. This is known as "inheritance." Knowing whether other family members have previously had this disease, also known as "family health history," can be very important information for the medical team.

Autosomal Dominant

Autosomal means the gene involved is located on one of the numbered chromosomes. Dominant means that a child only needs to inherit one copy of the mutated gene from either biological parent to be affected by the disease. People affected by an autosomal dominant disease have a 50 percent chance of passing on the mutated gene to their biological child.

Autosomal Recessive

Autosomal means the gene involved is located on one of the numbered chromosomes. Recessive means that a child must inherit two copies of the mutated gene, one from each biological parent, to be affected by the disease. A carrier is a person who only has one copy of the genetic mutation. A carrier usually does not show any symptoms of the disease. If both biological parents are carriers, there is a 25 percent chance their child inherits both copies of the mutated gene and is affected by the disease. Additionally, there is a 50 percent chance their child inherits only one copy of the mutated gene and is a carrier.

X-Linked

X-linked inheritance means the genetic mutation is located on the X chromosome, one of the sex chromosomes. The male sex chromosome pair consists of one X and one Y chromosome (XY). The female sex chromosome pair consists of two X chromosomes (XX). Because males have just one X chromosome, it takes only one copy of the mutated gene to cause the disease. Females that have one copy of the mutated gene may have symptoms similar to those experienced by affected males but usually have less severe symptoms or no symptoms at all. Female parents with one X-linked mutated gene have a 50 percent chance of passing on the mutation to each of their biological children. Male parents with an X-linked mutated gene will pass on the mutation to all their female children but cannot pass the mutation on to their male children.

HOW CAN PATIENT ORGANIZATIONS HELP?

Patient organizations can help people and families connect. They build public awareness of the disease and are a driving force behind research to improve patients' lives. They may offer online and in-person resources to help people live well with their disease. Many collaborate with medical experts and researchers.

Services of patient organizations differ but may include:

- ways to connect to others and share personal stories
- easy-to-read information
- up-to-date treatment and research information
- patient registries
- lists of specialists or specialty centers
- financial aid and travel resources[1]

---

[1] Genetic and Rare Diseases Information Center (GARD) "Nephrogenic Diabetes Insipidus," National Center for Advancing Translational Sciences (NCATS), August 2024. Available online. URL: https://rarediseases.info.nih.gov/diseases/7178/nephrogenic-diabetes-insipidus. Accessed October 22, 2024.

Chapter 13 | **Kidney and Renal Pelvis Cancer**

The body has two kidneys, one on each side, located behind the liver and stomach. The kidneys make urine, which is how the body washes liquid waste out of the body. The kidneys also control blood pressure and stimulate the bone marrow to make red blood cells. The renal pelvis is in the center of the kidney and is responsible for collecting the urine and feeding it into the ureters, two tubes that connect the kidneys with the bladder. The bladder holds urine until it leaves the body.

Kidney and renal pelvis cancer is a disease in which cells in the kidney grow out of control. It can also be called "renal cell cancer," as that is the most common type of kidney and renal pelvis cancer.

SYMPTOMS

A person with kidney or renal pelvis cancer may or may not have one or more of the following symptoms. The same symptoms can also arise from other causes. If any of these symptoms occur, consultation with a doctor is advised:

- blood in the urine
- a lump or swelling in the kidney area or abdomen
- lower back pain or pain in the side that does not go away
- feeling tired often
- fever that keeps coming back
- not feeling like eating
- losing weight for no reason that is known
- something blocking the bowels
- a general feeling of poor health

RISK FACTORS

Risk factors for kidney and renal pelvis cancers include:

- being overweight or having obesity
- smoking
- having high blood pressure (HBP). It is not known whether the increased risk is due to high blood pressure itself or the medicines used to treat it
- taking certain pain medicines for a long time
- having certain genetic conditions
- having a long-lasting infection with hepatitis C
- having kidney stones
- having sickle cell trait, which is associated with a very rare form of kidney cancer (renal medullary carcinoma)
- being exposed to a chemical called "trichloroethylene," which is used to remove grease from metal

REDUCING RISK

To lower the risk of kidney and renal pelvis cancers, consider the following recommendations:

- Do not smoke, or quit if currently smoking.
- Maintain a healthy weight.
- Eat a healthy diet.
- Be physically active.
- Be very careful when using certain chemicals, especially trichloroethylene, which is used by workers in some jobs, such as those that work with metals.[1]

DIAGNOSIS

Tests that examine the abdomen and kidneys are used to diagnose renal cell cancer. In addition to asking about personal and family

[1] "Kidney Cancer Basics," Centers for Disease Control and Prevention (CDC), November 6, 2023. Available online. URL: www.cdc.gov/kidney-cancer/about. Accessed October 22, 2024.

health history and conducting a physical exam, a doctor may perform the following tests and procedures:

- **Ultrasound exam.** This test uses high-energy sound waves (ultrasound) that bounce off internal tissues or organs and create echoes. The echoes form a picture of body tissues called a "sonogram."
- **Blood chemistry study.** This test uses a blood sample to measure the amounts of certain substances released into the blood by organs and tissues in the body. An unusual (higher or lower than normal) amount of a substance can be a sign of disease.
- **Urinalysis.** This test checks the color of urine and its contents, such as sugar, protein, red blood cells, and white blood cells.
- **CT scan (CAT scan).** This test uses a computer linked to an x-ray machine to create a series of detailed pictures of areas inside the body, such as the abdomen and pelvis. The pictures are taken from different angles and are used to create 3D views of tissues and organs. A dye may be injected into a vein or swallowed to help the organs or tissues show up more clearly. This procedure is also called "computed tomography," "computerized tomography," or "computerized axial tomography."
- **MRI (magnetic resonance imaging).** This test uses a magnet, radio waves, and a computer to create a series of detailed pictures of areas inside the body. This procedure is also called "nuclear magnetic resonance imaging" (NMRI).
- **Biopsy.** This procedure involves removing cells or tissues so they can be viewed under a microscope by a pathologist to check for signs of cancer. To perform a biopsy for renal cell cancer, a thin needle is inserted into the tumor, and a sample of tissue is withdrawn. A biopsy may not be needed if the imaging test results provide enough information to make a diagnosis.

After renal cell cancer has been diagnosed, tests are performed to find out if cancer cells have spread within the kidney or to other parts of the body. The process used to find out if cancer has spread within the kidney or to other parts of the body is called "staging." The information gathered from the staging process determines the stage of the disease. It is important to know the stage in order to plan treatment.

Some tests and procedures used to diagnose renal cell cancer, such as CT scan and MRI, may also be used in the staging process. Other tests include the following:

- **Chest x-ray**. This type of radiation can go through the body and create pictures of organs and bones inside the chest.
- **Bone scan**. This procedure checks if there are rapidly dividing cells, such as cancer cells, in the bone. A very small amount of radioactive material is injected into a vein and travels through the bloodstream. The radioactive material collects in the bones with cancer and is detected by a scanner.

Some people decide to get a second opinion. Seeking a second opinion can confirm the renal cell cancer diagnosis and treatment plan. If a second opinion is pursued, it is necessary to obtain medical test results and reports from the first doctor to share with the second doctor. The second doctor will review the pathology report, slides, and scans. They may agree with the first doctor, suggest changes or another treatment approach, or provide more information about the cancer.

STAGES

The following stages are used for renal cell cancer:

- stage I renal cell cancer
- stage II renal cell cancer
- stage III renal cell cancer
- stage IV renal cell cancer

Renal cell cancer can recur (come back) many years after initial treatment. The cancer stage describes the extent of cancer in the body, such as the size of the tumor, whether it has spread, and how far it has spread from where it first formed.

Several staging systems for cancer describe the extent of the cancer. Renal cell cancer staging usually uses the TNM Classification of Malignant Tumors (TNM) staging system, which may be described in the pathology report. Based on the TNM results, a stage (I, II, III, or IV) is assigned to the cancer. When discussing the diagnosis, a doctor may describe the cancer as one of these stages.

TREATMENT OPTIONS

Different types of treatments are available for people with renal cell cancer. The cancer care team will work together to decide the treatment plan, which may include more than one type of treatment. Many factors will be considered, such as the stage of the cancer, overall health, and preferences. The plan will include information about the cancer, the goals of treatment, treatment options, possible side effects, and the expected length of treatment.

The following types of treatment are used:

- surgery
- radiation therapy
- immunotherapy
- targeted therapy

FOLLOW-UP CARE

As treatment progresses, follow-up tests or check-ups will be necessary. Some tests that were performed to diagnose or stage the cancer may be repeated to assess the effectiveness of the treatment. The results of these tests may be used to decide whether to continue, change, or stop treatment.

Some tests will continue to be conducted periodically after treatment has ended. The results of these tests can indicate if the condition has changed or if the cancer has recurred (come back).

After treatment for renal cell cancer, a blood test to measure amounts of carcinoembryonic antigen (a substance in the blood that may be increased when cancer is present) may be performed to assess if the cancer has returned.[2]

---

[2] "Renal Cell Cancer Treatment (PDQ®)–Patient Version," National Cancer Institute (NCI), October 11, 2024. Available online. URL: www.cancer.gov/types/kidney/patient/kidney-treatment-pdq. Accessed October 22, 2024.

Chapter 14 | Renal Tubular Acidosis

WHAT IS RENAL TUBULAR ACIDOSIS?

Renal tubular acidosis (RTA) occurs when the kidneys do not remove acids from the blood into the urine as they should. The acid level in the blood then becomes too high, a condition called "acidosis." Some acid in the blood is normal, but too much acid can disturb many bodily functions.

There are three main types of RTA:

1. Type 1 RTA or distal RTA occurs when there is a problem at the end or distal part of the tubules.
2. Type 2 RTA or proximal RTA occurs when there is a problem in the beginning or proximal part of the tubules.
3. Type 4 RTA or hyperkalemic RTA occurs when the tubules are unable to remove enough potassium, which also interferes with the kidney's ability to remove acid from the blood.

Type 3 RTA is rarely used as a classification now because it is thought to be a combination of type 1 and type 2 RTA.

HOW COMMON IS RENAL TUBULAR ACIDOSIS?

Renal tubular acidosis is a rare disease that is often misdiagnosed or undiagnosed, making it difficult to determine the true frequency in the general population.

WHO IS MORE LIKELY TO HAVE RENAL TUBULAR ACIDOSIS?

People are more likely to have type 1 RTA if they inherit specific genes from their parents or if they have certain autoimmune diseases such as Sjögren syndrome or lupus.

People with Fanconi syndrome or those taking medicines to treat HIV or viral hepatitis are more likely to have type 2 RTA. People who inherit genes for type 2 RTA from their parents may also have it. In adults, type 2 RTA can be a complication or side effect of multiple myeloma, exposure to toxins, or certain medications. In rare cases, type 2 RTA occurs in people who experience chronic rejection of a transplanted kidney.

People with low levels of the hormone aldosterone, those who cannot urinate freely because of an obstruction, or those who have had a kidney transplant are more likely to develop type 4 RTA. One in five people develop type 4 RTA if they experience rejection of a transplanted kidney or are taking immunosuppressive medications.

WHAT ARE THE COMPLICATIONS OF RENAL TUBULAR ACIDOSIS?

Type 1 Renal Tubular Acidosis

Untreated type 1 RTA causes children to grow more slowly and adults to develop progressive kidney disease and bone diseases. Adults and children with untreated type 1 RTA may develop kidney stones because of abnormal calcium deposits that build up in the kidneys. These deposits prevent the kidneys from working properly.

Other diseases and conditions related to type 1 RTA include:

- a hereditary form of deafness
- renal medullary cystic disease
- sickle cell anemia
- Ehlers-Danlos syndrome
- urinary tract infections

Type 2 Renal Tubular Acidosis

Untreated type 2 RTA may cause children to grow more slowly. In addition, it may cause rickets—a bone disease—and dental disease in both children and adults. A very low potassium level can develop during the treatment of type 2 RTA with alkali.

Type 4 Renal Tubular Acidosis

In people with type 4 RTA, high levels of potassium in the blood can lead to muscle weakness or heart problems, such as slow or irregular heartbeats and cardiac arrest.

WHAT ARE THE SIGNS AND SYMPTOMS OF RENAL TUBULAR ACIDOSIS?

The major signs of type 1 and type 2 RTA are low blood levels of potassium and bicarbonate, a waste product produced by the body. The potassium level drops if the kidneys send too much potassium into the urine instead of returning it to the blood.

Because potassium helps regulate nerve and muscle health and heart rate, low potassium levels can cause:

- extreme weakness
- irregular heartbeat
- paralysis
- death

The major signs of type 4 RTA are high potassium and low bicarbonate levels in the blood. Symptoms of type 4 RTA include:

- abdominal pain
- fatigue that does not go away
- weak muscles
- not feeling hungry
- weight change

WHAT ARE THE CAUSES OF RENAL TUBULAR ACIDOSIS?

Type 1 Renal Tubular Acidosis

Type 1 RTA may be inherited. Researchers have identified at least three different genes that may cause the inherited form of the disease. People with sickle cell anemia or Ehlers-Danlos syndrome, which is also inherited, may develop type 1 RTA later in life.

However, type 1 RTA may develop because of an autoimmune disease, such as Sjögren syndrome or lupus, that can affect many parts of the body. These diseases may interfere with the removal of acid from the blood.

Type 1 RTA can also be caused by certain medications, including some used for pain and bipolar disorder, conditions causing high calcium in the urine, blocked urinary tract, or rejection of a transplanted kidney.

Type 2 Renal Tubular Acidosis

Type 2 RTA may be inherited or caused by other inherited conditions such as:

- cystinosis, a rare disease in which cystine crystals are deposited in bones and other tissues
- hereditary fructose intolerance
- Wilson disease

Type 2 RTA can also be caused by acute lead poisoning or chronic exposure to cadmium. It can also occur in people treated with certain medications used in chemotherapy and to treat HIV, viral hepatitis, glaucoma, migraines, and seizures.

Type 2 RTA almost always occurs as part of Fanconi syndrome. The main features of Fanconi syndrome include:

- abnormal excretion of glucose, amino acids, citrate, bicarbonate, and phosphate into the urine
- low blood potassium levels
- low levels of vitamin D

Type 4 Renal Tubular Acidosis

Type 4 RTA can occur when blood levels of the hormone aldosterone are low or when the kidneys do not respond to the hormone. Aldosterone directs the kidneys to regulate the sodium level, which also affects the levels of chloride and potassium in the blood.

Certain medications that interfere with the kidneys' task of moving electrolytes between blood and urine may also cause type 4 RTA. Some of these include:

- blood pressure medicines—angiotensin-converting enzyme (ACE) inhibitors and angiotensin receptor blockers (ARBs)

- certain diuretics used to treat congestive heart failure that do not decrease potassium in the blood
- certain medications to prevent blood from clotting
- some immunosuppressive medications that prevent the rejection of transplanted organs
- painkillers—nonsteroidal anti-inflammatory drugs (NSAIDs)
- antibiotics used to treat pneumonia, urinary tract infections, and traveler's diarrhea

Type 4 RTA can also occur when diseases or an inherited disorder affect how the kidneys work, such as:

- Addison disease, due to disease or removal of the adrenal glands
- congenital adrenal insufficiency
- aldosterone synthase deficiency
- Gordon syndrome
- amyloidosis
- diabetic kidney disease
- HIV/AIDS
- kidney transplant rejection
- lupus
- sickle cell disease
- urinary tract obstruction

HOW DO HEALTH-CARE PROFESSIONALS DIAGNOSE RENAL TUBULAR ACIDOSIS?

A health-care professional will review medical history and order blood and urine tests to measure the levels of acid, base, and potassium in the blood and urine. If the blood is more acidic than it should be and the urine is less acidic than it should be, RTA may be the reason, but a health-care professional will need to rule out other causes.

If RTA is diagnosed, information about the sodium, potassium, and chloride levels in the urine and the potassium level in the blood will help identify which type of RTA is present.

HOW DO HEALTH-CARE PROFESSIONALS TREAT RENAL TUBULAR ACIDOSIS?

For all types of RTA, drinking a solution of sodium bicarbonate or sodium citrate will lower the acid level in the blood. This alkali therapy can prevent kidney stones from forming and help the kidneys function more normally, preventing worsening kidney failure.

Infants with type 1 RTA may need potassium supplements, but older children and adults rarely do because alkali therapy prevents the kidneys from excreting potassium into the urine.

Children with type 2 RTA will also drink an alkali solution (sodium bicarbonate or potassium citrate) to lower the acid level in their blood, prevent bone disorders and kidney stones, and grow normally. Some adults with type 2 RTA may need to take vitamin D supplements to help prevent bone problems.

People with type 4 RTA may need other medicines to lower potassium levels in the blood.

If RTA is caused by another condition, a health-care professional will attempt to identify and treat it.[1]

[1] "Renal Tubular Acidosis," National Institute of Diabetes and Digestive and Kidney Diseases (NIDDK), November 2020. Available online. URL: www.niddk.nih.gov/health-information/kidney-disease/renal-tubular-acidosis. Accessed October 22, 2024.

Part 3 | Disorders of the Urinary Tract

Chapter 15 | Understanding Urinary Tract Infections

Chapter Contents

Section 15.1 | Overview of Urinary Tract Infections

Do you have pain or burning when you urinate? You might have a urinary tract infection (UTI). Antibiotics treat UTIs. Your healthcare provider can determine if you have a UTI and what antibiotic you need.

The urinary tract includes the bladder, urethra, and kidneys. UTIs are common infections that happen when bacteria, often from the skin or rectum, enter the urethra and infect the urinary tract.

TYPES AND STRAINS OF URINARY TRACT INFECTIONS

- bladder infection (most common, also known as "cystitis")
- kidney infection (less common but more serious, also known as "pyelonephritis")

SIGNS AND SYMPTOMS OF URINARY TRACT INFECTIONS

Symptoms of a bladder infection can include:

- pain or burning while urinating
- frequent urination
- feeling the need to urinate despite having an empty bladder
- bloody urine
- pressure or cramping in the groin or lower abdomen

Symptoms of a kidney infection can include:

- fever
- chills
- lower back pain or pain in the side of your back
- nausea or vomiting

Younger children may not be able to tell you about the UTI symptoms they are having. While fever is the most common sign of a UTI in infants and toddlers, most children with fever do not have a UTI.

WHEN TO SEEK MEDICAL CARE

If you or your child have symptoms of a UTI or any symptom that is severe or concerning, talk to your health-care provider right away. If your child is younger than three months old and has a fever of 100.4 °F (38 °C) or higher, seek medical care immediately.

RISK FACTORS OF URINARY TRACT INFECTIONS

Urinary tract infections are more common in females because their urethras are shorter and closer to the rectum, making it easier for bacteria to enter the urinary tract.

Other risk factors include:

- a previous UTI
- recent sexual activity
- changes in the bacteria that live inside the vagina or vaginal flora. For example, menopause or the use of spermicides can cause these bacterial changes
- pregnancy
- age (older adults and young children are more likely to get UTIs)
- structural problems in the urinary tract, such as an enlarged prostate
- poor hygiene, for example, in children who are potty-training

PREVENTION OF URINARY TRACT INFECTIONS

- Urinate after sexual activity.
- Stay well hydrated.
- Take showers instead of baths.
- Minimize douching, sprays, or powders in the genital area.
- Teach girls, when potty training, to wipe front to back.

DIAGNOSIS OF URINARY TRACT INFECTIONS

Your health-care provider will determine if you have a UTI by:

- asking about symptoms
- doing a physical exam
- ordering urine tests, if needed
- starting an antibiotic to treat a UTI, if needed

TREATMENT OF URINARY TRACT INFECTIONS

Taking antibiotics prescribed by a health-care provider can treat most UTIs. Your health-care provider might also recommend medicine to help lessen the pain or discomfort. Some cases may require treatment in a hospital.

Any time you take antibiotics, they can cause side effects.

Side effects can include rash, dizziness, nausea, diarrhea, and yeast infections. More serious side effects can include antimicrobial-resistant infections or *Clostridioides difficile* infection, which causes diarrhea that can lead to severe colon damage and death.

Call your health-care provider if you develop any side effects while taking your antibiotic.

HOW TO FEEL BETTER

- Drink plenty of water or other fluids.
- If your health-care provider prescribes you antibiotics:
  - Take antibiotics exactly as your health-care provider tells you.
  - Do not share your antibiotics with others.
  - Do not save antibiotics for later. Talk to your health-care provider about safely discarding leftover antibiotics.[1]

Section 15.2 | **Bladder Infections (Urinary Tract Infections) in Adults**

WHAT IS A BLADDER INFECTION?

A bladder infection is an illness most often caused by bacteria that enter the bladder and multiply. It is the most common type of urinary tract infection (UTI). If untreated, bladder infections can spread to the kidneys and develop into a more serious infection.

[1] "Urinary Tract Infection Basics," Centers for Disease Control and Prevention (CDC), January 22, 2024. Available online. URL: www.cdc.gov/uti/about/index.html. Accessed October 17, 2024.

Bladder infections may also be called "cystitis."

Sometimes, people use the more general term UTI to refer to bladder infections. However, UTIs can occur in other parts of the urinary tract, including the urethra and kidneys.

HOW COMMON ARE BLADDER INFECTIONS?

Bladder infections are more common in women than in men. Research shows that about half of all women will develop a bladder infection in their lifetime. About a quarter of those women will have repeat infections. Men under age 50 rarely get bladder infections.

WHO IS MORE LIKELY TO DEVELOP A BLADDER INFECTION?

Females are more likely to develop bladder infections than males due to their anatomy. Females have a short urethra located close to the anus, a source of bacteria. Therefore, bacteria from the anus may more easily enter the female urinary tract and cause a bladder infection. However, anyone with a bladder can develop a bladder infection, including children.

You are more likely to develop a bladder infection if you:

- are sexually active or have gone through menopause
- use certain types of birth control, such as a diaphragm or spermicide
- had a UTI in the past
- have difficulty emptying your bladder completely
- use, or have recently used, a urinary catheter
- have a urinary tract blockage, such as a kidney stone or enlarged prostate
- have an abnormality in the urinary tract, such as vesicoureteral reflux
- have diabetes or problems with your immune system

WHAT ARE THE COMPLICATIONS OF A BLADDER INFECTION?

When diagnosed early and treated properly, most bladder infections do not lead to complications. If untreated, a bladder infection can spread to one or both kidneys. Kidney infections are often very painful. Without treatment, kidney infections can cause serious health problems, such as permanent kidney damage.

Bladder infections that occur during pregnancy are more likely to spread to the kidneys. If you are pregnant, your health-care professional may test your urine for bacteria. Regular testing can help your health-care professional diagnose and treat a bladder infection before it leads to complications.

WHAT ARE THE SYMPTOMS OF A BLADDER INFECTION?

Symptoms of a bladder infection may include:

- a burning feeling when you urinate
- frequent or intense urges to urinate, even when you have little urine to pass
- pain or discomfort in the lower abdomen
- cloudy, bloody, or strong-smelling urine

WHEN SHOULD I SEEK A HEALTH-CARE PROFESSIONAL'S HELP?

Contact a health-care professional if you have symptoms of a bladder infection.

Bladder infections can spread to one or both kidneys. Quick treatment is important if you have symptoms of a kidney infection, such as:

- fever and chills
- nausea or vomiting
- pain in your back, side, or groin

Kidney infections may cause severe pain and serious health problems if not treated early.

WHAT CAUSES A BLADDER INFECTION?

Bladder infections are most often caused by bacteria. Rarely, fungi may cause a bladder infection.

Normally, the body keeps bacteria in the urinary tract in balance. Emptying your bladder, or urinating, is one way the body helps maintain a healthy number of bacteria in the bladder.

DIAGNOSIS OF BLADDER INFECTION IN ADULTS

Health-care professionals use your medical history, a physical exam, and lab tests to diagnose a bladder infection. In some cases, a health-care professional may use other tests to help find the cause of a bladder infection. Health-care professionals may use lab tests to test your urine or blood. Lab tests include urinalysis, urine culture, and blood tests. Your health-care professional may also use imaging or other tests.

TREATMENT FOR BLADDER INFECTION IN ADULTS

If you have a bladder infection caused by bacteria, your health-care professional will likely prescribe antibiotics. However, you can help speed up your recovery and ease your symptoms by drinking more liquids, which helps flush the bacteria out of your urinary tract.

Your health-care professional may also prescribe over-the-counter pain relievers to help with pain. You may be asked to use medicine such as ibuprofen or acetaminophen.

Sometimes, your health-care professional cannot confirm a diagnosis based on symptoms and test results. You may not need antibiotics. Instead, your health-care professional will work to find the cause and another way to treat your symptoms.

HOW CAN I PREVENT A BLADDER INFECTION?

Sometimes, you may be able to help prevent a bladder infection by taking the steps below.

Keep Your Urinary Tract Healthy

You can help keep your urinary tract healthy by:

- drinking enough liquids
- developing healthy bathroom habits, including wiping front to back
- using the bathroom when you feel the urge to urinate
- taking the time to fully empty your bladder when urinating

Wear Loose-Fitting Clothing

Consider wearing cotton underwear and loose-fitting clothes that do not trap moisture. Some health-care professionals think that too much moisture increases the risk of infection.

Consider Switching Birth Control Methods

Talk with your health-care professional about switching your birth control if you have repeat bladder infections. Some forms of birth control, such as diaphragms, unlubricated condoms, or spermicide, may increase your chances of getting a bladder infection.

Consider Using Vaginal Estrogen

If you are in perimenopause or menopause and you have repeat bladder infections, your health-care professional may prescribe low-dose vaginal estrogen. Vaginal estrogen increases good bacteria and helps prevent infection.[1]

Section 15.3 | **Bladder Infections (Urinary Tract Infections) in Children**

WHAT IS A BLADDER INFECTION?

A bladder infection is an illness that is usually caused by bacteria. Bladder infections are the most common type of urinary tract infection (UTI) in children. A UTI can develop in any part of your child's urinary tract, including the urethra, bladder, ureters, or kidneys.

All healthy children have some bacteria on their bodies and in their bowels. Occasionally, bacteria can get into the bladder and start an infection. Children of any age, including infants, can and do develop bladder infections.

---

[1] "Bladder Infection (Urinary Tract Infection—UTI) in Adults," National Institute of Diabetes and Digestive and Kidney Diseases (NIDDK), April 2024. Available online. URL: www.niddk.nih.gov/health-information/urologic-diseases/bladder-infection-uti-in-adults. Accessed October 17, 2024.

Your child's body has ways to defend against infection. For example, urine normally flows from your child's kidneys, through the ureters, to the bladder. Bacteria that enter the urinary tract are flushed out when your child urinates. This one-way flow of urine keeps bacteria from infecting the urinary tract. Sometimes the body's defenses fail, and the bacteria cause a bladder infection. If your child has symptoms of a bladder infection or has a fever without a clear cause, see a health-care professional within 24 hours.

Bladder infections are also called "cystitis."

Sometimes, people use the more general term UTI to mean a bladder infection, although UTIs can occur in other parts of the urinary system. A UTI that affects the kidneys is called "pyelonephritis."

HOW COMMON ARE BLADDER INFECTIONS IN CHILDREN?

Bladder infections are a common reason that children visit a health-care professional. Each year, about 3 in 100 children develop a UTI, and most of these infections are bladder infections.

- Babies under 12 months old are more likely to have a UTI than older children.
- During the first few months of life, UTIs are more common in boys than in girls.
- By age one, girls are more likely to develop a UTI than boys—and girls continue to have a higher risk throughout childhood and the teen years.

WHICH CHILDREN ARE MORE LIKELY TO DEVELOP A BLADDER INFECTION?

Girls are much more likely to develop bladder infections than boys, except during the first year of life. Among boys younger than age one, those who have not had the foreskin of the penis removed, called a "circumcision," have a higher risk for a bladder infection. Still, most uncircumcised boys will not get a bladder infection.

In general, any condition or habit that keeps urine in your child's bladder for too long may lead to an infection.

Other factors that may make your child more likely to develop a bladder infection include:

- abnormal bladder function or habits, such as:
  - overactive bladder—a treatable condition that often goes away as your child grows older
  - not emptying the bladder fully
  - waiting too long to urinate
  - constipation—fewer than two bowel movements a week or hard bowel movements that are painful or difficult to pass
- vesicoureteral reflux (VUR)—the backward flow of some urine from the bladder toward the kidneys during urination
- urinary blockage—a problem that limits the normal flow of urine, such as a kidney stone or a ureter that is too narrow. In some cases, this can be related to a birth defect
- poor toilet hygiene
- family history of UTIs

Among teen girls, those who are sexually active are more likely to get a bladder infection.

Different anatomy makes girls much more likely to develop a bladder infection than boys:

- Girls have a shorter urethra than boys, so bacteria do not have to go as far to reach the bladder and cause an infection.
- In girls, the urethra is closer to the anus, a source of bacteria that can cause a bladder infection.

WHAT ARE THE COMPLICATIONS OF BLADDER INFECTIONS IN CHILDREN?

Quick treatment is likely to cure your child's bladder infection with no complications.

If an infection in the lower urinary tract, such as a bladder infection, is not treated properly, it can lead to a kidney infection. Kidney infections that last a long time or keep coming back can cause damage to a child's kidneys that never goes away. This damage can include kidney scars, poor kidney function, high blood pressure (HBP), and problems during pregnancy. Young children have a greater risk for kidney damage from a UTI than older children and adults.

In a few cases, a kidney infection can develop suddenly and become life-threatening, particularly if bacteria get into the bloodstream, causing a reaction called "sepsis" or "septicemia."

WHAT ARE THE SYMPTOMS OF A BLADDER INFECTION?

Do not assume that you will know when your child has a bladder infection, even if you have had one yourself. Symptoms can be very different in children than in adults, especially for infants and preschoolers. If your child is not well, contact your child's pediatrician or health clinic.

Young Children

It is not always obvious when an infant or child younger than age two has a bladder infection. Sometimes there are no symptoms, or your child may be too young to explain what feels wrong. A urine test is the only way to know for certain whether your child has a bladder or kidney infection.

When a young child has symptoms of a UTI, they may include:

- fever, which may be the only sign
- vomiting or diarrhea
- irritability or fussiness
- poor feeding or appetite; poor weight gain

Older Children

Symptoms of a bladder or kidney infection in a child ages two and older can include:

- pain or burning when urinating
- cloudy, dark, bloody, or foul-smelling urine
- frequent or intense urges to urinate
- pain in the lower belly area or back

- fever
- wetting after a child has been toilet trained

SEEK CARE RIGHT AWAY

If you think your child has a bladder infection, take him or her to a health-care professional within 24 hours. A child who has a high fever and is sick for more than a day without a runny nose, earache, or other obvious cause should also be checked for a bladder infection. Quick treatment is important to prevent the infection from becoming more dangerous.

WHAT CAUSES A BLADDER INFECTION?

Most often, a bladder infection is caused by bacteria that are normally found in the bowel. The bladder has several systems to prevent infection. For example, urinating most often flushes out bacteria before it reaches the bladder. Sometimes, your child's body cannot fight the bacteria, and the bacteria cause an infection. Certain health conditions can put children at risk for bladder infections.

HOW DO HEALTH-CARE PROFESSIONALS DIAGNOSE A BLADDER INFECTION?

Health-care professionals use your child's medical history, a physical exam, and tests to diagnose a bladder infection.

A health-care professional will ask about health conditions that may make your child more likely to develop a bladder infection.

During a physical exam, the health-care professional will also ask about your child's symptoms.

WHAT TESTS DO HEALTH-CARE PROFESSIONALS USE TO DIAGNOSE A BLADDER INFECTION?

Health-care professionals typically test a urine sample, called "urinalysis," to help diagnose a bladder infection. A urine culture, which takes longer to come back from the lab, is needed for an accurate diagnosis. In some cases, a health-care professional may order more tests to look at your child's urinary tract.

Lab Tests

URINALYSIS

A small amount of your child's urine must be collected for this test. Babies and small children who are not toilet trained will have a small, thin, flexible tube called a "catheter" placed into the urethra to get a urine sample. This is needed because urine from collection bags, which can be taped around a baby's diaper area, is often contaminated or mixed with germs and other substances found on the baby's skin. If urine is contaminated, test results will not be accurate.

Parents may help preschoolers catch a clean urine sample in a special container, and older children and teens can do it by themselves.

A health-care professional will look at the sample under a microscope for bacteria and white blood cells, which the body produces to fight infection. Bacteria also can be found in the urine of healthy children, so a bladder infection is diagnosed based on both your child's symptoms and lab test results.

URINE CULTURE

A health-care professional must order a urine culture to find out what type of bacteria is causing your child's infection. Lab workers will monitor how the bacteria multiply, usually over one to three days, to help determine the best treatment for your child.

Imaging Tests

A health-care professional may order imaging tests to find the cause of your child's infection or to check for kidney damage.

ULTRASOUND

An ultrasound uses specialized sound waves to look at structures inside the body without exposing your child to radiation. During this painless test, your child lies on a padded table. A technician gently moves a wand called a "transducer" over your child's belly and back. Ultrasound can create images of your child's entire urinary tract. No anesthesia is needed.

Ultrasound may be recommended if your child:

- is younger than age two and has a bladder infection with a fever
- has had repeated bladder infections at any age
- has high blood pressure, poor growth, or a family history of kidney or bladder problems
- does not get better with treatment

An ultrasound may be scheduled right away or a few weeks or months after your child's illness has passed.

VOIDING CYSTOURETHROGRAM

A voiding cystourethrogram (VCUG) uses x-rays of the bladder and urethra to show how urine flows. A catheter is used to fill your child's bladder with a special dye. Then, x-ray pictures are taken before and after your child urinates. A VCUG can show if urine flows backward from the bladder into the ureters or kidneys, a condition called "vesicoureteral reflux" (VUR). Anesthesia is not needed for this test, but your child may be offered a calming medicine, called a "sedative."

HOW DO HEALTH-CARE PROFESSIONALS TREAT BLADDER INFECTIONS IN CHILDREN?

Bladder infections in children are treated with antibiotics, a type of medicine that fights bacteria.

Medicines

Which antibiotic your child takes depends on age, allergies to antibiotics, and the type of bacteria causing the UTI. Children older than two months usually take an antibiotic by mouth—as a liquid or as a chewable tablet.

Your child may go to a hospital for intravenous (IV) antibiotics if the child is younger than two months old or vomiting. IV medicines are given through a vein.

Your child should start to feel better within a day or two, but it is important to take every dose of the antibiotic on time and to finish all the medicine. The infection could come back if your child stops taking the antibiotic too soon.

The length of treatment depends on:

- how severe the infection is
- whether a child's symptoms and infection go away
- whether a child has repeated bladder infections
- whether the child has vesicoureteral reflux or another problem in the urinary tract

At-Home Treatments

Children should drink plenty of liquids and urinate often to speed healing. Drinking water is best. Ask your health-care professional how much liquid your child should drink.

A heating pad on a child's back or abdomen may help ease pain from a kidney or bladder infection.

HOW CAN YOU HELP YOUR CHILD PREVENT A BLADDER INFECTION?

Drinking enough liquids, following good bathroom and diapering habits, wearing loose-fitting clothes, and getting treated for related health problems may help prevent a UTI in a child or teen.

Be Sure Your Child Drinks Enough Liquids

Drinking more liquids may help flush bacteria from the urinary tract. Talk with a health-care professional about how much liquid your child should drink and which beverages are best to help prevent a repeat UTI.

Follow Good Bathroom and Diapering Habits

Some children simply do not urinate often enough. Children should urinate often and when they first feel the need to go. Bacteria can grow and cause an infection when urine stays in the bladder too long. Caregivers should change diapers often for infants and toddlers and should clean the genital area well. Gentle cleansers that do not irritate the skin are best.

Your child should always wipe from front to back after urinating or having a bowel movement. This step is most important after a bowel movement to keep bacteria from getting into the urethra and bladder.

Avoid Constipation

Hard stools can press against the urinary tract and block the flow of urine, allowing bacteria to grow. Helping your child have regular bowel movements can prevent constipation.

Wear Loose-Fitting Clothing

Consider having children wear cotton underwear and loose-fitting clothes so air can keep the area around the urethra dry.

Treat Related Health Problems

When a child's bladder does not work exactly as it should—called "dysfunctional voiding"—treatments may help the bladder work better and prevent repeated infections. The muscles that control urination may be out of sync, or your child's bladder may be overactive or underactive.

Health-care professionals can treat these types of bladder problems with medicines, behavior changes, or both. Children often grow out of these bladder problems naturally over time.

If your child has vesicoureteral reflux, a urinary tract blockage, or an anatomical problem, see a pediatric urologist or other specialist. Treating these conditions may help prevent repeated bladder infections.

Diabetes and other health conditions can increase the risk of a bladder infection. Ask your child's health-care professional how to reduce the risk of developing a bladder infection.[1]

---

[1] "Bladder Infection (Urinary Tract Infection—UTI) in Children," National Institute of Diabetes and Digestive and Kidney Diseases (NIDDK), April 2017. Available online. URL: www.niddk.nih.gov/health-information/urologic-diseases/urinary-tract-infections-in-children. Accessed October 17, 2024.

Section 15.4 | **Urinary Tract Infections during Pregnancy**

WHAT ARE URINARY TRACT INFECTIONS?

Urinary tract infections (UTIs) are most often caused by bacteria (germs) that get into the bladder, which is part of the urinary tract. UTIs are also called "bladder infections." UTIs are common, especially in women. More than half of women will have at least one UTI at some point in life. UTIs are serious and often painful. However, most UTIs are easy to treat with antibiotics. UTIs can happen anywhere in the urinary system (which includes the kidneys, ureters, bladder, and urethra). UTIs are most common in the bladder. A UTI in the bladder is called "cystitis." Infections in the bladder can spread to the upper part of the urinary tract or the kidneys. A UTI in the kidneys is called "pyelonephritis" or "pyelo."

Women get UTIs up to 30 times more often than men do. Additionally, as many as 4 in 10 women who get a UTI will get at least one more within six months.

Women get UTIs more often because a woman's urethra (the tube from the bladder to where the urine exits the body) is shorter than a man's. This makes it easier for bacteria to get into the bladder. A woman's urethral opening is also closer to both the vagina and the anus, the main sources of germs such as *Escherichia coli* (*E. coli*) that cause UTIs.

UTIs are most often caused by bacteria that enter the urinary tract, leading to infections primarily in the bladder. Infections can spread to the upper urinary tract, including the kidneys, potentially causing more serious health concerns.

RISK FACTORS FOR URINARY TRACT INFECTIONS

You may be at greater risk for a UTI if you:

- are sexually active, as sexual activity can transfer germs that cause UTIs from other areas, such as the vagina, to the urethra
- use a diaphragm for birth control or spermicides with a diaphragm or condoms, which can kill good bacteria that protect against UTIs

- are pregnant, since pregnancy hormones can alter the bacteria in the urinary tract and increase the likelihood of UTIs
- have gone through menopause, which leads to a loss of estrogen causing vaginal tissue to become thin and dry, thereby facilitating the growth of harmful bacteria
- have diabetes, which can weaken your immune system and cause nerve damage that makes it difficult to empty your bladder fully
- have any condition that obstructs urine flow, such as a kidney stone, which can increase your risk of UTIs
- have or recently had a catheter in place, as catheters can introduce bacteria into the bladder, especially during surgical procedures when you cannot pass urine independently

COMMON SYMPTOMS OF URINARY TRACT INFECTIONS

If you have a UTI, you may experience some or all of the following symptoms:

- pain or burning when urinating
- an urge to urinate often, but not much comes out when you go
- pressure in your lower abdomen
- urine that smells bad or looks milky or cloudy
- blood in the urine (This is more common in younger women. If you see blood in your urine, tell a doctor or nurse right away.)
- feeling tired, shaky, confused, or weak (This is more common in older women.)
- having a fever, which may mean the infection has reached your kidneys

POTENTIAL RISKS OF UNTREATED URINARY TRACT INFECTIONS IN PREGNANCY

If treated right away, a UTI is not likely to damage your urinary tract. However, if left untreated, the infection can spread to the kidneys and other parts of your body. The most common symptoms of a kidney infection are fever and pain in the back where the kidneys are located. Antibiotics can also treat kidney infections.

Sometimes, the infection can enter the bloodstream, which is rare but life-threatening. Changes in hormone levels during pregnancy raise the risk for UTIs, which are more likely to spread to the kidneys.

If you are pregnant and have symptoms of a UTI, see your doctor or nurse right away. Your doctor will prescribe an antibiotic that is safe to take during pregnancy.

If left untreated, UTIs could lead to kidney infections and problems during pregnancy, including:

- premature birth (birth of the baby before 39–40 weeks)
- low birth weight (smaller than 5.5 pounds at birth)
- high blood pressure (HBP), which can lead to a more serious condition called "preeclampsia"

Women who get two UTIs in six months or three in a year have recurrent UTIs. Your doctor or nurse might perform tests to find out why. If the test results are normal, you may need to take a small dose of antibiotics every day to prevent infection. Your doctor may also provide a supply of antibiotics to take after sex or at the first sign of infection.[1]

[1] Office on Women's Health (OWH), "Urinary Tract Infections," U.S. Department of Health and Human Services (HHS), February 22, 2021. Available online. URL: www.womenshealth.gov/a-z-topics/urinary-tract-infections. Accessed October 17, 2024.

Chapter 16 | Kidney Stones

Chapter Contents

Section 16.1 | Understanding Kidney Stones

Each year, more than 1 million people in the United States rush to the emergency room with pain caused by a kidney stone.

Kidney stones are hard, pebble-like pieces of material that form in one or both kidneys. They are caused by high levels of certain minerals in the urine.

Stones vary in size from tiny crystals that can only be seen with a microscope to stones over an inch wide. Tiny stones may pass out of the body without the person even noticing, but with larger stones, this is not the case. Stones larger than a pencil eraser can get stuck in the urinary tract, which can be extremely painful.

Everyone is at some risk of developing kidney stones. Kidney stones can form at any age, but they usually appear during middle age (40s–60s). Of those who develop one stone, half will develop at least one more in the future.

During the warmest months of the year, the risk of dehydration increases, making it necessary to drink plenty of water to help prevent kidney stones.

DIAGNOSIS OF KIDNEY STONES

A doctor may order lab or imaging tests to detect kidney stones. Lab tests analyze urine for blood, signs of infection, minerals (such as calcium), and stones. Blood tests can also detect high levels of certain minerals. Knowing what the stones are made of can help guide treatment.

Imaging tests, such as CT scans or plain x-rays, can help the doctor pinpoint the location and estimate the size of a kidney stone. Depending on the findings, the doctor may prescribe medication and advise drinking plenty of fluids. In some cases, a procedure may be necessary to break up or remove the kidney stone.

TREATMENT OPTIONS

There are different procedures for breaking up or removing kidney stones. One method delivers shock waves to the stone from outside the body. Other strategies involve inserting a tool into the body, either through the urinary tract or directly into the kidney through surgery. After locating the stone, it can be broken up into smaller pieces.

WHEN TO SEEK MEDICAL ATTENTION

See a health-care provider if you experience:

- sharp, severe pains in the back, side, lower belly, or groin
- nausea and vomiting
- blood in the urine, which may appear pink, red, or brown
- constant need to empty the bladder
- pain when urinating
- difficulty urinating

Once you have had a kidney stone, you have an increased chance of having another. Do not let the pain of kidney stones send you to the emergency room; keep hydrated![1]

Section 16.2 | **Kidney Stones in Children**

WHAT ARE KIDNEY STONES?

Kidney stones are hard, pebble-like pieces of material that form in one or both of a child's kidneys when high levels of certain minerals occur in urine (see Figure 16.1). If treated by a health-care professional, kidney stones rarely cause permanent damage.

Kidney stones vary in size and shape. They may be as small as a grain of sand or as large as a pea. Rarely, some kidney stones are as large as golf balls. Kidney stones may be smooth or jagged and are usually yellow or brown.

---

[1] *NIH News in Health*, "Pebbles in Your Plumbing," National Institutes of Health (NIH), June 2017. Available online. URL: https://newsinhealth.nih.gov/2017/06/pebbles-your-plumbing. Accessed October 16, 2024.

A small kidney stone may pass through the urinary tract on its own, causing little or no pain. A larger kidney stone may get stuck along the way. A kidney stone that gets stuck can block the flow of urine, causing severe pain or bleeding.

A child who has symptoms of kidney stones, including severe pain, blood in the urine, or vomiting, needs care right away. A health-care professional, such as a urologist, can treat any pain and determine how and when to treat the kidney stone. The provider may also prescribe medicine to prevent further problems or treat a urinary tract infection (UTI).

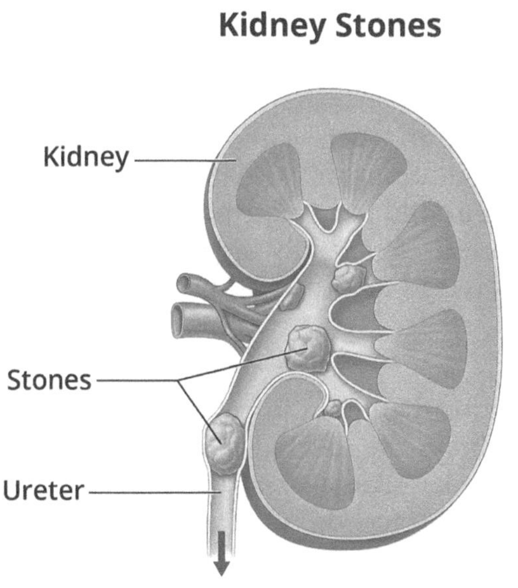

Figure 16.1. Kidney Stones

National Institute of Diabetes and Digestive and Kidney Diseases (NIDDK)

DO KIDNEY STONES HAVE ANOTHER NAME?

The scientific name for a kidney stone is "renal calculus" or "nephrolith." Health-care professionals may refer to this condition as "nephrolithiasis," "urolithiasis," or "urinary stones."

WHAT TYPES OF KIDNEY STONES OCCUR IN CHILDREN?

Children develop one of four main types of kidney stones.

Calcium Stones

Calcium stones, including calcium oxalate stones and calcium phosphate stones, are the most common types of kidney stones in children. Calcium oxalate stones are more prevalent than calcium phosphate stones.

Calcium from food does not increase the chance of having calcium oxalate stones. Normally, calcium that is not taken up by a child's bones and muscles goes to the kidneys and is flushed out with urine. In some children, the kidneys leak extra calcium, which can join with other waste products to form a kidney stone.

Uric Acid Stones

A uric acid stone may form when a child's urine contains too much uric acid. Medical conditions or inherited disorders can lead to excessive uric acid in a child's urinary tract. Less often, consuming fish, shellfish, and meat—especially organ meats—may increase uric acid in urine and lead to kidney stones.

Struvite Stones

Struvite stones may form after an infection in the upper urinary tract, where the kidneys are located. These stones can develop suddenly and become large quickly. Struvite stones tend to affect children whose urinary tracts did not develop normally, causing limited or blocked urine flow. Simple UTIs, such as bladder infections, usually do not lead to struvite stones.

Cystine Stones

Cystine stones result from a disorder called "cystinuria" that is passed down through families. In cystinuria, a child's kidneys leak large amounts of cysteine, an amino acid. Cystine crystals can then form in the urine and cause stones.

Treatment for kidney stones usually depends on their size, location, and composition.

HOW COMMON ARE KIDNEY STONES IN CHILDREN?

Kidney stones are not common in children, but the number of affected children has steadily increased over the last several years. Changing eating habits may be responsible, especially the rise in sodium consumption through processed foods and table salt. The increase in obesity and less active lifestyles may also contribute to a higher incidence of kidney stones among children.

WHICH CHILDREN ARE MORE LIKELY TO DEVELOP KIDNEY STONES?

Children of all ages can develop kidney stones, including infants, but they occur much more often in teenagers. A family history of kidney stones makes a child more likely to develop them. Children who have had kidney stones in the past have a greater chance of developing another kidney stone.

An unhealthy lifestyle and diet can increase the likelihood of kidney stones. For example, drinking too little water or consuming inappropriate liquids, such as sugary soft drinks or drinks with caffeine, may cause substances in the urine to become too concentrated.

Likewise, excessive sodium, a component of salt, may force extra minerals into the urine, potentially leading to kidney stones. Unhealthy amounts of sodium are found in many prepared foods, including restaurant meals, chips, sandwich meats, frozen foods, and some sports drinks.

Children with Certain Conditions

Children are more likely to develop kidney stones if they have certain conditions, including:

- a blockage in or abnormal shape of the urinary tract
- chronic, or long-lasting, inflammation of the bowel
- cystic fibrosis
- cystic kidney diseases—disorders that cause fluid-filled sacs to form on the kidneys
- cystinuria
- digestive problems or a history of gastrointestinal tract surgery

- gout—a disorder that causes painful swelling of the joints
- hypercalciuria—a condition that runs in families in which urine contains unusually large amounts of calcium; this is the most common condition found in people who form calcium stones
- hyperoxaluria—a condition in which urine contains unusually large amounts of oxalate
- hyperparathyroidism—a condition in which the parathyroid glands release too much parathyroid hormone, causing extra calcium in the blood
- hyperuricosuria—a disorder in which too much uric acid is in the urine
- obesity
- repeated UTIs
- renal tubular acidosis—a disease that occurs when the kidneys fail to remove acids into the urine, causing a person's blood to remain too acidic

Children Who Take Certain Medicines

Children are more likely to develop kidney stones when taking the following medicines or medicinal diets over a long period of time:

- diuretics, often called "water pills"—medications used to rid the body of excess water
- calcium-based antacids
- excessive vitamin D
- indinavir and other protease inhibitors—medications used to treat HIV infection
- topiramate and zonisamide—medications used for seizures and migraine headaches
- ketogenic diet—a diet used for seizure disorders that do not respond to medication

WHAT ARE THE COMPLICATIONS OF KIDNEY STONES IN CHILDREN?

Complications of kidney stones are rare if a child is treated by a health-care professional before problems occur.

If kidney stones are not treated, they can cause:

- hematuria, or blood in the urine
- severe pain
- UTIs, including kidney infections
- loss of kidney function[1]

Section 16.3 | Treatment and Prevention of Kidney Stones

Health-care professionals usually treat kidney stones based on their size, location, and type.

Small kidney stones may pass through the urinary tract without treatment. If a patient is able to pass a kidney stone, a health-care professional may ask them to collect it in a special container. The professional will then send the kidney stone to a lab to determine its type. The patient may be advised to drink plenty of liquids to help move the kidney stone along and may also receive a prescription for pain medication.

Larger kidney stones, or those that block the urinary tract or cause significant pain, may require urgent treatment. If a patient is vomiting and dehydrated, they may need to go to the hospital for intravenous (IV) fluids.

KIDNEY STONE REMOVAL

A urologist can remove kidney stones or break them into smaller pieces using the following treatments:

- **Shock wave lithotripsy**. This method uses shock waves to blast the kidney stone into smaller pieces, which can then pass through the urinary tract. Anesthesia is administered during this outpatient procedure.
- **Cystoscopy and ureteroscopy**. During cystoscopy, the doctor uses a cystoscope to look inside the urethra

[1] "Definition and Facts of Kidney Stones in Children," National Institute of Diabetes and Digestive and Kidney Diseases (NIDDK), May 2017. Available online. URL: www.niddk.nih.gov/health-information/urologic-diseases/kidney-stones-children/definition-facts. Accessed October 17, 2024.

and bladder to locate a stone. Ureteroscopy involves a ureteroscope, which is longer and thinner than a cystoscope, to view detailed images of the lining of the ureters and kidneys. The doctor inserts the cystoscope or ureteroscope through the urethra to examine the urinary tract. Once the stone is located, it can be removed or broken into smaller pieces. These procedures are performed in a hospital under anesthesia, and patients can typically go home the same day.

- **Percutaneous nephrolithotomy**. In this procedure, the doctor uses a thin viewing tool called a "nephroscope" to locate and remove the kidney stone. The nephroscope is inserted directly into the kidney through a small incision made in the back. For larger stones, the doctor may also use a laser to break the stones into smaller pieces. This procedure is conducted in a hospital with anesthesia, and patients may need to stay in the hospital for several days afterward.

After these procedures, the urologist may leave a thin, flexible tube called a "ureteral stent" in the urinary tract to facilitate urine flow or the passage of any remaining stone fragments. Once the kidney stone is removed, the doctor sends the stone or its pieces to a lab for analysis to determine its type.

The health-care professional may also ask the patient to collect urine for 24 hours after the kidney stone has passed or been removed. This allows for the measurement of daily urine production and mineral levels. Patients who do not produce enough urine each day or have high mineral levels are more likely to form stones.

HOW CAN YOU PREVENT KIDNEY STONES?

Identifying the cause of any previous kidney stones is essential to helping prevent future ones. Once the type of kidney stone is known, a health-care professional can assist in making dietary and lifestyle changes to prevent future occurrences.

Drinking Liquids

Drinking enough liquids each day is the best way to prevent most types of kidney stones. Adequate hydration keeps urine diluted and helps flush away minerals that might form stones.

While water is the best option, other liquids such as citrus drinks may also help prevent kidney stones. Some studies suggest that citrus drinks, such as lemonade and orange juice, protect against kidney stones due to their citrate content, which inhibits crystal formation.

Unless kidney failure is present, individuals should aim to drink six to eight 8-ounce glasses of water daily. Those with cystine stones may need to increase their fluid intake. It is advisable to consult a health-care professional if you are unable to meet these fluid intake recommendations due to other health issues, such as urinary incontinence or kidney failure.

The amount of liquid required can vary based on weather and activity level. Hot weather or exercise may necessitate increased fluid intake to replace fluids lost through sweat. A health-care professional may request a 24-hour urine collection to determine daily urine volume. If urine output is insufficient, the professional may recommend increasing liquid consumption.

Medications

For individuals who have had kidney stones, a health-care professional may prescribe medications to help prevent future stones. The type of medication prescribed will depend on the type of kidney stone and may need to be taken for several weeks or longer.

For example, if struvite stones are present, an oral antibiotic may be prescribed for one to six weeks or longer.

For other types of stones, potassium citrate may be prescribed to be taken one to three times daily. Patients may need to continue potassium citrate for months or longer until a health-care professional determines they are no longer at risk for kidney stones.

It is important to discuss health history with a health-care professional before starting kidney stone medications. Some medications may have side effects, which can be more pronounced with long-term use or higher doses. Report any side effects to your health-care professional.

Table 16.1 provides information on different types of kidney stones and the possible medications that may be prescribed by a doctor for each type.

Table 16.1. Commonly Prescribed Medications by Kidney Stone Type

Type of Kidney Stone	Medication Type
Calcium stones	• Potassium citrate, which is used to raise the citrate and pH levels in urine • Diuretics, often called "water pills," help rid your body of water
Uric acid stones	• Allopurinol, which is used to treat high levels of uric acid in the body • Potassium citrate
Struvite stones	• Antibiotics, which are bacteria-fighting medications • Acetohydroxamic acid, a strong antibiotic, used with another long-term antibiotic medication to prevent infection
Cystine stoncs	• Mercaptopropionyl glycine, an antioxidant used for heart problems • Potassium citrate

Hyperparathyroidism Surgery

People with hyperparathyroidism, a condition characterized by excess calcium in the blood, may develop calcium stones. Treatment for hyperparathyroidism may involve surgery to remove the abnormal parathyroid gland. Successfully removing the parathyroid gland can cure hyperparathyroidism and help prevent kidney stones, though surgery may carry some risks, including infection.[1]

[1] "Treatment for Kidney Stones," National Institute of Diabetes and Digestive and Kidney Diseases (NIDDK), May 2017. Available online. URL: www.niddk.nih.gov/health-information/urologic-diseases/kidney-stones/treatment. Accessed October 17, 2024.

Section 16.4 | Managing Kidney Stone Risk through Diet

CAN I HELP PREVENT KIDNEY STONES BY CHANGING WHAT I EAT OR DRINK?

Drinking enough liquid, mainly water, is the most important thing you can do to prevent kidney stones. Unless you have kidney failure, many health-care professionals recommend that you drink six to eight 8-ounce glasses a day. Talk with a health-care professional about how much liquid you should drink.

Studies have shown that the Dietary Approaches to Stop Hypertension (DASH) diet can reduce the risk of kidney stones (www.nhlbi.nih.gov/education/dash-eating-plan).

Studies have shown that being overweight increases your risk of kidney stones. A dietitian can help you plan meals to help you lose weight.

DOES THE TYPE OF KIDNEY STONE I HAD AFFECT FOOD CHOICES I SHOULD MAKE?

Yes. If you have already had kidney stones, ask your health-care professional which type of kidney stone you had. Based on the type of kidney stone you had, you may be able to prevent kidney stones by making changes in how much sodium, animal protein, calcium, or oxalate is in the food you eat.

You may need to change what you eat and drink for these types of kidney stones:

- calcium oxalate stones
- calcium phosphate stones
- uric acid stones
- cystine stones

A dietitian who specializes in kidney stone prevention can help you plan meals to prevent kidney stones. Find a dietitian who can help you.

Calcium Oxalate Stones

REDUCE OXALATE

If you have had calcium oxalate stones, you may want to avoid these foods to help reduce the amount of oxalate in your urine:

- nuts and nut products
- peanuts—which are legumes, not nuts, and are high in oxalate
- rhubarb
- spinach
- wheat bran

Talk with a health-care professional about other food sources of oxalate and how much oxalate should be in your diet.

REDUCE SODIUM

Your chance of developing kidney stones increases when you eat more sodium. Sodium is a part of salt. Sodium is in many canned, packaged, and fast foods. It is also in many condiments, seasonings, and meats.

Talk with a health-care professional about how much sodium should be in what you eat.

LIMIT ANIMAL PROTEIN

Eating animal protein may increase your chances of developing kidney stones.

A health-care professional may tell you to limit eating animal protein, including:

- beef, chicken, and pork, especially organ meats
- eggs
- fish and shellfish
- milk, cheese, and other dairy products

Although you may need to limit how much animal protein you eat each day, you still need to ensure you get enough. Consider replacing some of the meat and animal protein you would typically eat with beans, dried peas, and lentils, which are plant-based foods that are high in protein and low in oxalate.

Talk with a health-care professional about how much total protein you should eat and how much should come from animal or plant-based foods.

GET ENOUGH CALCIUM FROM FOODS

Even though calcium sounds like it would be the cause of calcium stones, it is not. In the right amounts, calcium can block other substances in the digestive tract that may lead to stones. Talk with a health-care professional about how much calcium you should eat to help prevent getting more calcium oxalate stones and to support strong bones. It may be best to get calcium from low-oxalate, plant-based foods such as calcium-fortified juices, cereals, breads, some kinds of vegetables, and some types of beans. Ask a dietitian or other health-care professional which foods are the best sources of calcium for you.

Calcium Phosphate Stones

REDUCE SODIUM

Your chance of developing kidney stones increases when you eat more sodium. Sodium is a part of salt. Sodium is in many canned, packaged, and fast foods. It is also in many condiments, seasonings, and meats.

Talk with a health-care professional about how much sodium should be in what you eat.

LIMIT ANIMAL PROTEIN

Eating animal protein may increase your chances of developing kidney stones.

A health-care professional may tell you to limit eating animal protein, including:

- beef, chicken, and pork, especially organ meats
- eggs
- fish and shellfish
- milk, cheese, and other dairy products

Although you may need to limit how much animal protein you have each day, you still need to make sure you get enough protein.

Consider replacing some of the meat and animal protein you would typically eat with some of these plant-based foods that are high in protein:

- legumes such as beans, dried peas, lentils, and peanuts
- soy foods, such as soy milk, soy nut butter, and tofu
- nuts and nut products, such as almonds and almond butter, cashews and cashew butter, walnuts, and pistachios
- sunflower seeds

Talk with a health-care professional about how much total protein you should eat and how much should come from animal or plant-based foods.

GET ENOUGH CALCIUM FROM FOODS

Even though calcium sounds like it would be the cause of calcium stones, it is not. In the right amounts, calcium can block other substances in the digestive tract that may lead to stones. Talk with a health-care professional about how much calcium you should eat to help prevent getting more calcium phosphate stones and to support strong bones. It may be best to get calcium from plant-based foods such as calcium-fortified juices, cereals, breads, some kinds of vegetables, and some types of beans. Ask a dietitian or other health-care professional which foods are the best sources of calcium for you.

Uric Acid Stones

LIMIT ANIMAL PROTEIN

Eating animal protein may increase your chances of developing kidney stones.

A health-care professional may tell you to limit eating animal protein, including:

- beef, chicken, and pork, especially organ meats
- eggs
- fish and shellfish
- milk, cheese, and other dairy products

Although you may need to limit how much animal protein you have each day, you still need to make sure you get enough protein. Consider replacing some of the meat and animal protein you would typically eat with some of these plant-based foods that are high in protein:

- legumes such as beans, dried peas, lentils, and peanuts
- soy foods, such as soy milk, soy nut butter, and tofu
- nuts and nut products, such as almonds and almond butter, cashews and cashew butter, walnuts, and pistachios
- sunflower seeds

Talk with a health-care professional about how much total protein you should eat and how much should come from animal or plant-based foods.

Losing weight if you are overweight is especially important for people who have had uric acid stones.

Cystine Stones

Drinking enough liquid, mainly water, is the most important lifestyle change you can make to prevent cystine stones. Talk with a health-care professional about how much liquid you should drink.[1]

[1] "Eating, Diet, and Nutrition for Kidney Stones," National Institute of Diabetes and Digestive and Kidney Diseases (NIDDK), May 2017. Available online. URL: www.niddk.nih.gov/health-information/urologic-diseases/kidney-stones/eating-diet-nutrition. Accessed October 17, 2024.

Chapter 17 | **Congenital Genital and Urinary Disorders in Newborns**

Chapter Contents

Section 17.1 | Hypospadias

WHAT IS HYPOSPADIAS?

Hypospadias occurs when the opening of the urethra is not located at the tip of the penis. The urethra is the tube that carries urine from the bladder to the outside of the body.

In boys with hypospadias, the urethra forms abnormally during weeks 8–14 of pregnancy. The abnormal opening can form anywhere from just below the end of the penis to the scrotum.

Boys with hypospadias can sometimes have a curved penis. They may experience problems with abnormal spraying of urine and might need to sit to urinate. In some boys with hypospadias, the testicle has not fully descended into the scrotum. If hypospadias is not treated, it can lead to complications later in life, including difficulty performing sexual intercourse or difficulty urinating while standing.

TYPES OF HYPOSPADIAS

The types of hypospadias depend on the location of the opening of the urethra:

- **Subcoronal.** The opening of the urethra is located somewhere near the head of the penis.
- **Midshaft.** The opening of the urethra is located along the shaft of the penis.
- **Penoscrotal.** The opening of the urethra is located where the penis and scrotum meet.

RISK FACTORS OF HYPOSPADIAS

The causes of hypospadias in most infants are unknown. The Centers for Disease Control and Prevention (CDC) researchers have reported findings about some factors that affect the risk of having a baby with hypospadias, including:

- maternal age of 30 years or older
- maternal body mass index (BMI) classified as overweight or obese

- use of assisted reproductive technology to conceive
- maternal use of certain hormones (progestins) just before or during pregnancy

DIAGNOSIS OF HYPOSPADIAS

Hypospadias is usually diagnosed during a physical examination after the baby is born.

TREATMENT OF HYPOSPADIAS

The treatment for hypospadias depends on the type of defect the boy has. Most cases require surgery to correct the defect.

If surgery is needed, it is typically performed when the boy is between the ages of 3 and 18 months. In some cases, the surgery is done in stages. Some of the repairs performed during the surgery might include:

- placing the opening of the urethra in the correct position
- correcting the curve in the penis
- repairing the skin around the opening of the urethra

The doctor may need to use the foreskin to perform some of the repairs. This means a baby boy with hypospadias should not be circumcised.[1]

Section 17.2 | **Urine Blockage**

WHAT IS THE URINARY TRACT?

The urinary tract is the body's drainage system for removing wastes and extra fluid. The urinary tract includes two kidneys, two ureters, a bladder, and a urethra. The kidneys are two bean-shaped organs, each about the size of a fist. They are located just below

[1] "Hypospadias," Centers for Disease Control and Prevention (CDC), May 16, 2024. Available online. URL: www.cdc.gov/birth-defects/about/hypospadias.html. Accessed October 17, 2024.

the rib cage, one on each side of the spine. Every day, the kidneys filter about 120–150 quarts of blood to produce about 1–2 quarts of urine, composed of wastes and extra fluid. Children produce less urine than adults, and the amount produced depends on their age. The urine flows from the kidneys to the bladder through tubes called "ureters." The bladder stores urine until it is released through urination. When the bladder empties, urine flows out of the body through a tube called the "urethra" at the bottom of the bladder.

The kidneys and urinary system keep fluids and natural chemicals in the body balanced. While a baby is developing in the mother's womb, known as "prenatal development," the placenta—a temporary organ joining mother and baby—controls much of that balance. The baby's kidneys begin to produce urine at about 10–12 weeks after conception. However, the mother's placenta continues to do most of the work until the last few weeks of the pregnancy. Wastes and extra water are removed from the baby's body through the umbilical cord. The baby's urine is released into the amniotic sac and becomes part of the amniotic fluid. This fluid plays a role in the baby's lung development.

WHAT CAUSES URINE BLOCKAGE IN NEWBORNS?

Many types of defects in the urinary tract can cause urine blockage:

- **Vesicoureteral reflux (VUR).** Most children with VUR are born with a ureter that did not grow long enough during development in the womb. The valve formed by the ureter pressing against the bladder wall does not close properly, so urine backs up—refluxes—from the bladder to the ureter and eventually to the kidney. Severe reflux may prevent a kidney from developing normally and may increase the risk of damage from infections after birth. VUR usually affects only one ureter and kidney, though it can affect both ureters and kidneys.
- **Ureteropelvic junction (UPJ) obstruction.** If urine is blocked where the ureter joins the kidney, only the kidney swells. The ureter remains a normal size. UPJ obstruction usually occurs in only one kidney.

- **Bladder outlet obstruction (BOO).** BOO describes any blockage in the urethra or at the opening of the bladder. Posterior urethral valves (PUV), the most common form of BOO seen in newborns and during prenatal ultrasound exams, is a birth defect in boys in which an abnormal fold of tissue in the urethra keeps urine from flowing freely out of the bladder. This defect may cause swelling in the entire urinary tract, including the urethra, bladder, ureters, and kidneys.
- **Ureterocele.** If the end of the ureter does not develop normally, it can bulge, creating a ureterocele. The ureterocele may obstruct part of the ureter or the bladder.

Some babies are born with genetic conditions that affect several different systems in the body, including the urinary tract:

- **Prune belly syndrome (PBS).** PBS is a group of birth defects involving poor development of the abdominal muscles, enlargement of the ureters and bladder, and both testicles remaining inside the body instead of descending into the scrotum. The skin over the abdomen is wrinkled, giving the appearance of a prune. PBS usually occurs in boys, and most children with PBS have hydronephrosis—swelling in the kidney—and VUR.
- **Esophageal atresia (EA).** EA is a birth defect in which the esophagus—the muscular tube that carries food and liquids from the mouth to the stomach—lacks the opening for food to pass into the stomach. Babies born with EA may also have problems with their spinal columns, digestive systems, hearts, and urinary tracts.
- **Congenital heart defects.** Heart defects range from mild to life-threatening. Children born with heart defects also have a higher rate of problems in the urinary tract than children in the general population, suggesting that some types of heart and urinary defects may have a common genetic cause.

Urine blockage can also be caused by spina bifida and other birth defects that affect the spinal cord. These defects may interrupt nerve signals between the bladder, spinal cord, and brain, which are needed for urination. In newborns, urinary retention—the inability to empty the bladder completely—can lead to urinary retention. Urine that remains in the bladder can reflux into the ureters and kidneys, causing swelling.

WHAT ARE THE SYMPTOMS OF URINE BLOCKAGE IN NEWBORNS?

Before leaving the hospital, a baby with urine blockage may urinate only small amounts or may not urinate at all. As part of the routine newborn exam, the health-care provider may feel an enlarged kidney or find a closed urethra, which may indicate urine blockage. Sometimes urine blockage is not apparent until a child develops symptoms of a urinary tract infection (UTI), including:

- fever
- irritability
- not eating
- nausea
- diarrhea
- vomiting
- cloudy, dark, bloody, or foul-smelling urine
- urinating often

If these symptoms persist, the child should see a health-care provider. A child two months of age or younger with a fever should see a health-care provider immediately. The provider will ask for a urine sample to test for bacteria.

WHAT ARE THE COMPLICATIONS OF URINE BLOCKAGE BEFORE AND AFTER BIRTH?

When a defect in the urinary tract blocks the flow of urine, the urine backs up and causes the ureters to swell, a condition called "hydroureter" and "hydronephrosis."

Hydronephrosis is the most common problem found during prenatal ultrasound of a baby in the womb. The swelling may be easy to see or barely detectable. The results of hydronephrosis may be mild or severe, yet the long-term outcome for the child's health cannot always be predicted by the severity of swelling. Urine blockage may damage the developing kidneys and reduce their ability to filter. In the most severe cases of urine blockage, where little or no urine leaves the baby's bladder, the amount of amniotic fluid is reduced to the point that the baby's lung development is threatened.

After birth, urine blockage may raise a child's risk of developing a UTI. Recurring UTIs can lead to more permanent kidney damage.

HOW IS URINE BLOCKAGE IN NEWBORNS DIAGNOSED?

Defects of the urinary tract may be diagnosed before or after the baby is born.

Diagnosis before Birth

Tests during pregnancy can help determine if the baby is developing normally in the womb.

- **Ultrasound**. Ultrasound uses a device called a "transducer" that bounces safe, painless sound waves off organs to create an image of their structure. A prenatal ultrasound can show internal organs within the baby. The procedure is performed in a health-care provider's office, outpatient center, or hospital by a specially trained technician, and the images are interpreted by a radiologist—a doctor who specializes in medical imaging—or an obstetrician—a doctor who delivers babies. The images can show enlarged kidneys, ureters, or bladders in babies.
- **Amniocentesis**. It is a procedure in which amniotic fluid is removed from the mother's womb for testing. The procedure can be performed in the health-care provider's office, and local anesthetic may be used. The health-care provider inserts a thin needle through the abdomen into the uterus to obtain a small amount of amniotic fluid. Cells from the fluid are grown in a lab

and then analyzed. The health-care provider usually uses ultrasound to find the exact location of the baby. The test can show whether the baby has certain birth defects and how well the baby's lungs are developing.

- **Chorionic villus sampling (CVS).** CVS is the removal of a small piece of tissue from the placenta for testing. The procedure can be performed in the health-care provider's office; anesthesia is not needed. The health-care provider uses ultrasound to guide a thin tube or needle through the vagina or abdomen into the placenta. Cells are removed from the placenta and then analyzed. The test can show whether the baby has certain genetic defects.

Most healthy women do not need all of these tests. Ultrasound exams during pregnancy are routine. Amniocentesis and CVS are recommended only when a risk of genetic problems exists because of family history or when a problem is detected during an ultrasound. Amniocentesis and CVS carry a slight risk of harming the baby and mother or ending the pregnancy in miscarriage, so the risks should be carefully considered.

Diagnosis before Birth

Different imaging techniques can be used in infants and children to determine the cause of urine blockage.

- **Ultrasound.** Ultrasound can be used to view the child's urinary tract. For infants, the image is clearer than could be achieved while the baby was in the womb.
- **Voiding cystourethrogram (VCUG).** VCUG is an x-ray image of the bladder and urethra taken while the bladder is full and during urination, also called "voiding." The procedure is performed in an outpatient center or hospital by an x-ray technician supervised by a radiologist, who then interprets the images. While anesthesia is not needed, sedation may be used for some children. The bladder and urethra are filled with a special dye called "contrast medium" to make the

structures clearly visible on the x-ray images. The x-ray machine captures images of the contrast medium while the bladder is full and when the child urinates. The test can show reflux or blockage of the bladder due to an obstruction, such as PUV.

- **Radionuclide scan**. A radionuclide scan is an imaging technique that detects small amounts of radiation after a person is injected with radioactive chemicals. The dose of the radioactive chemicals is small; therefore, the risk of causing damage to cells is low. Radionuclide scans are performed in an outpatient center or hospital by a specially trained technician, and the images are interpreted by a radiologist. Anesthesia is not needed. Special cameras and computers are used to create images of the radioactive chemicals as they pass through the kidneys. Radioactive chemicals injected into the blood can provide information about kidney function.

HOW IS URINE BLOCKAGE IN NEWBORNS TREATED?

Treatment for urine blockage depends on the cause and severity of the blockage. Hydronephrosis discovered before the baby is born rarely requires immediate action, especially if it is only on one side. The condition often goes away without any treatment before or after birth. The health-care provider should keep track of the condition with frequent ultrasounds.

Surgery

If the urine blockage threatens the life of the unborn baby, a fetal surgeon may recommend surgery to insert a shunt or correct the problem causing the blockage. A shunt is a small tube that can be inserted into the baby's bladder to release urine into the amniotic sac. The procedure is similar to amniocentesis in that a needle is inserted through the mother's abdomen. Ultrasound guides the placement of the shunt, which is attached to the end of the needle. Alternatively, an endoscope—a small, flexible tube with a light—can be used to place a shunt or to repair the problem causing the blockage. Fetal surgery carries many risks, so it is performed only in special circumstances, such as when the amniotic fluid is absent and the baby's lungs are not developing or when the kidneys are severely damaged.

If the urinary defect does not correct itself after the child is born, and the child continues to have urine blockage, surgery may be needed to remove the obstruction and restore urine flow. The decision to operate depends on the degree of blockage. After surgery, a small tube, called a "stent," may be placed in the ureter or urethra to keep it open temporarily while healing occurs.

Antibiotics

Antibiotics are bacteria-fighting medications. A child with possible urine blockage or VUR may be given antibiotics to prevent UTIs from developing until the urinary defect corrects itself or is corrected with surgery.

Intermittent Catheterization

Intermittent catheterization may be used for a child with urinary retention due to a nerve disease. The parent or guardian, and later the child, is taught to drain the bladder by inserting a thin tube, called a "catheter," through the urethra to the bladder. Emptying the bladder in this way helps to decrease kidney damage, urine leakage, and UTIs.[1]

Section 17.3 | Hydronephrosis

WHAT IS HYDRONEPHROSIS IN NEWBORNS?

Hydronephrosis in newborns is the enlargement, or dilation, of the renal pelvis—the basin in the central part of the kidney where urine collects. Hydronephrosis can occur in one or both kidneys. This condition is often diagnosed before birth during a prenatal ultrasound.

In some cases, hydronephrosis is mild and resolves on its own without treatment. In other cases, it may indicate a blockage in the

[1] "Urine Blockage in Newborns," National Institute of Diabetes and Digestive and Kidney Diseases (NIDDK), September 15, 2013. Available online. URL: www.niddk.nih.gov/-/media/Files/Urologic-Diseases/UrineBlockage_508.pdf. Accessed October 17, 2024.

urinary tract or reflux—or backup—of urine from the bladder to the kidney that requires treatment.

The urinary tract is the body's drainage system for removing wastes and excess fluid. It includes the kidneys, ureters, bladder, and urethra.

HOW COMMON IS HYDRONEPHROSIS IN NEWBORNS?

In 1 or 2 out of every 100 pregnancies, the fetus is diagnosed with hydronephrosis. In about half of these cases, the hydronephrosis resolves by the time the infant is born.

WHO IS MORE LIKELY TO HAVE HYDRONEPHROSIS?

Males are about twice as likely as females to have hydronephrosis.

WHAT ARE THE SIGNS OR SYMPTOMS OF HYDRONEPHROSIS IN A NEWBORN?

Newborns with hydronephrosis often do not show signs. In some newborns, the abdomen may be swollen due to severe blockage of the urinary tract. In other cases, newborns with hydronephrosis may develop a urinary tract infection (UTI), which may cause signs or symptoms.

If your child has been diagnosed with hydronephrosis, talk with your child's health-care professional about appropriate evaluation and treatment options.

WHAT CAUSES HYDRONEPHROSIS IN NEWBORNS?

In some fetuses and newborns with hydronephrosis, health-care professionals cannot identify a cause, and the hydronephrosis resolves on its own. This is called "transient hydronephrosis."

In other cases, hydronephrosis is caused by a blockage in the urinary tract or reflux of urine from the bladder to the kidney.

Transient Hydronephrosis

Experts believe that the narrowing of part of the urinary tract during early development may cause transient hydronephrosis, which resolves as the urinary tract matures.

About half of fetuses diagnosed with hydronephrosis have transient hydronephrosis, which typically resolves before birth. In children born with hydronephrosis, the condition may be transient and can resolve on its own, usually by the age of three.

Birth Defects

Birth defects in the urinary tract may cause hydronephrosis. Even when birth defects are the cause, hydronephrosis may be mild and improve as the child grows. However, birth defects may also cause severe hydronephrosis or worsen over time.

URETER DEFECTS

Birth defects in the ureter that can cause hydronephrosis include:

- ureteropelvic junction (UPJ) obstruction, in which a blockage is present where the ureter joins the renal pelvis
- vesicoureteral reflux (VUR), in which urine flows backward, or refluxes, from the bladder to one or both ureters and sometimes to the kidneys
- other defects of the ureter or where the ureter joins the bladder, which may prevent the normal flow of urine from the kidneys to the bladder

Among all birth defects that cause hydronephrosis in fetuses and newborns, UPJ obstruction and VUR are the most common.

LOWER URINARY TRACT OBSTRUCTION

Lower urinary tract obstruction, also called "bladder outlet obstruction," occurs when a blockage is present in the urethra or where the bladder joins the urethra. Birth defects that cause lower urinary tract obstruction include posterior urethral valves, which are abnormal folds of tissue that block the urethra. Posterior urethral valves occur only in males. Because lower urinary tract obstruction blocks urine flow from both kidneys, it is more urgent for doctors to examine lower urinary tract obstruction than blockage or reflux in a ureter.

DEFECTS IN THE URINARY TRACT AND OTHER PARTS OF THE BODY

Some infants with hydronephrosis have birth defects in the urinary tract and in other parts of their body. For example, prune belly syndrome is a group of birth defects that includes poorly developed abdominal muscles, undescended testicles, and urinary tract defects.

Birth defects affecting the spinal cord, such as spina bifida, can influence the nerves controlling the urinary tract and cause urinary retention. Urine retained in the bladder may flow backward into the ureters and kidneys, causing hydronephrosis.

HOW DO HEALTH-CARE PROFESSIONALS DIAGNOSE HYDRONEPHROSIS BEFORE AN INFANT IS BORN?

Health-care professionals can diagnose hydronephrosis before an infant is born during a prenatal ultrasound. Ultrasound uses safe, painless sound waves to create an image of the fetus's organs. An ultrasound can reveal that parts of the urinary tract are enlarged due to hydronephrosis.

Ultrasounds during pregnancy are part of routine prenatal testing. If a fetus is diagnosed with hydronephrosis, health-care professionals may recommend additional ultrasounds to determine whether the condition worsens or improves over time. They may also use ultrasounds or other prenatal tests to try to find the cause of hydronephrosis or check for other health problems.

HOW DO HEALTH-CARE PROFESSIONALS DIAGNOSE HYDRONEPHROSIS IN NEWBORNS?

Health-care professionals diagnose hydronephrosis by examining a newborn's medical history, performing a physical exam, and performing imaging tests.

Medical History

Health-care professionals utilize the results of prenatal ultrasounds and other prenatal tests to determine what kind of testing or treatment infants will need after birth.

Physical Exam

During a physical exam, a health-care professional will check for a lump or mass in the abdomen, which could indicate an enlarged kidney or bladder. The professional will also check for signs of birth defects in other parts of the body.

Imaging Tests

Health-care professionals may use urinary tract imaging tests to diagnose and identify the cause of hydronephrosis. Imaging tests may include:

- ultrasound, which uses sound waves to visualize the child's urinary tract
- voiding cystourethrogram, which employs x-rays to show how urine flows through the bladder and urethra
- radionuclide scan, which creates images of the urinary tract as a radioactive substance passes through

HOW DO HEALTH-CARE PROFESSIONALS TREAT HYDRONEPHROSIS IN NEWBORNS?

Treatment of hydronephrosis in newborns will depend on:

- how severe the condition is
- whether one or both kidneys are affected
- what is causing the hydronephrosis

Treatments may include watchful waiting, preventing and treating UTIs and surgery.

Watchful Waiting

If hydronephrosis in a newborn is not severe and is not likely to damage the kidneys, health-care professionals may recommend watchful waiting. They will conduct tests periodically to assess whether hydronephrosis changes or causes kidney damage as the infant matures.

Hydronephrosis may improve or resolve over time. However, if hydronephrosis worsens or leads to complications, a health-care professional may recommend surgery.

Preventing and Treating Urinary Tract Infections

In some cases, health-care professionals may prescribe antibiotics to help prevent UTIs in infants and children with hydronephrosis. If a child develops a UTI, antibiotics are also utilized to treat the infection.

Research suggests that, in male infants with hydronephrosis, circumcision may lower the likelihood of developing UTIs.

Surgery

If hydronephrosis is severe or worsens over time, health-care professionals may recommend surgery. Surgery can enhance the flow of urine and reduce the chance of complications or prevent complications from worsening.

Health-care professionals rarely perform surgery to treat hydronephrosis in a fetus while still in the womb. Fetal surgery carries many risks and is performed only in special cases.[1]

[1] "Hydronephrosis in Newborns," National Institute of Diabetes and Digestive and Kidney Diseases (NIDDK), October 2019. Available online. URL: www.niddk.nih.gov/health-information/urologic-diseases/hydronephrosis-newborns. Accessed October 17, 2024.

Chapter 18 | Urethral Cancer

WHAT IS URETHRAL CANCER?

Urethral cancer is a disease in which malignant (cancer) cells form in the tissues of the urethra. The urethra is the tube that carries urine from the bladder to the outside of the body. In women, the urethra is about 1½ inches long and is situated just above the vagina. In men, the urethra is about 8 inches long and passes through the prostate gland and the penis to the outside of the body. In men, the urethra also carries semen.

Urethral cancer is a rare cancer that occurs more frequently in men than in women.

TYPES OF URETHRAL CANCER

There are different types of urethral cancer that begin in cells lining the urethra. These cancers are named for the types of cells that become malignant (cancerous):

- **Squamous cell carcinoma.** This is the most common type of urethral cancer. It forms in the thin, flat cells in the part of the urethra near the bladder in women and in the lining of the urethra in the penis in men.
- **Transitional cell carcinoma.** This type forms in the area near the urethral opening in women and in the part of the urethra that passes through the prostate gland in men.
- **Adenocarcinoma.** This type forms in the glands surrounding the urethra in both men and women.

Urethral cancer can metastasize (spread) quickly to tissues around the urethra and is often found in nearby lymph nodes by the time it is diagnosed.

RISK FACTORS FOR URETHRAL CANCER

A history of bladder cancer can affect the risk of urethral cancer. Anything that increases your chance of getting a disease is called a "risk factor." Having a risk factor does not mean that you will get cancer; not having risk factors does not guarantee that you will not get cancer. Talk with your doctor if you think you may be at risk. Risk factors for urethral cancer include the following:

- Having a history of bladder cancer.
- Having conditions that cause chronic inflammation in the urethra, including:
    - sexually transmitted diseases (STDs), including human papillomavirus (HPV), especially HPV type 16
    - frequent urinary tract infections (UTIs)

SIGNS AND SYMPTOMS OF URETHRAL CANCER

Signs of urethral cancer include bleeding or trouble with urination. These and other signs and symptoms may be caused by urethral cancer or by other conditions. There may be no signs or symptoms in the early stages. Check with your doctor if you have:

- trouble starting the flow of urine
- weak or interrupted ("stop-and-go") flow of urine
- frequent urination, especially at night
- incontinence
- discharge from the urethra
- bleeding from the urethra or blood in the urine
- a lump or thickness in the perineum or penis
- a painless lump or swelling in the groin

DIAGNOSIS OF URETHRAL CANCER

Tests that examine the urethra and bladder are used to diagnose urethral cancer. The following tests and procedures may be used:

- physical exam and health history
- pelvic exam
- digital rectal exam
- urine cytology
- urinalysis
- blood chemistry studies

- complete blood count (CBC)
- CT scan (CAT scan)
- ureteroscopy
- biopsy

PROGNOSIS AND TREATMENT OPTIONS FOR URETHRAL CANCER

Certain factors affect prognosis (chance of recovery) and treatment options. The prognosis and treatment options depend on:

- where the cancer formed in the urethra
- whether the cancer has spread through the mucosa lining the urethra to nearby tissue, to lymph nodes, or to other parts of the body
- whether the patient is male or female
- the patient's general health
- whether the cancer has just been diagnosed or has recurred (come back)

The following types of treatment are used:

- surgery
- radiation therapy
- chemotherapy

Some treatments are standard (the currently used treatment), and some are being tested in clinical trials. A treatment clinical trial is a research study meant to help improve current treatments or obtain information on new treatments for patients with cancer. When clinical trials show that a new treatment is better than the standard treatment, the new treatment may become the standard treatment. Patients may want to consider participating in a clinical trial. Some clinical trials are open only to patients who have not started treatment.

FOLLOW-UP TESTS

As you undergo treatment, you will have follow-up tests or check-ups. Some tests that were performed to diagnose or stage the cancer may be repeated to see how well the treatment is working. The results of these tests may be used to decide whether to continue, change, or stop treatment.

Some tests will continue to be performed periodically after treatment has ended. The results can show whether your condition has changed or if the cancer has recurred (come back).[1]

[1] "Urethral Cancer Treatment (PDQ®)–Patient Version," National Cancer Institute (NCI), October 7, 2022. Available online. URL: www.cancer.gov/types/urethral/patient/urethral-treatment-pdq. Accessed October 25, 2024.

Part 4 | Disorders of the Bladder and Prostate

Chapter 19 | Essential Steps for Maintaining Bladder Health

UNDERSTANDING BLADDER HEALTH

People rarely talk about bladder health, but everyone is affected by it. Located in the lower abdomen, the bladder is a hollow organ, much like a balloon, that stores urine. Urine contains waste and extra fluid left over after the body takes what it needs from what we eat and drink. Each day, adults pass about a quart and a half of urine through the bladder and out of the body.

As people age, their bladders change. The elastic bladder tissue may toughen and become less stretchy. A less flexible bladder cannot hold as much urine as before and might make you go to the bathroom more often. The bladder wall and pelvic floor muscles may weaken, making it harder to empty the bladder fully and causing urine to leak.

STEPS FOR MAINTAINING A HEALTHY BLADDER

- **Use the bathroom often and when needed.** Try to urinate at least once every three to four hours. Holding urine in your bladder for too long can weaken your bladder muscles and make a bladder infection more likely.
- **Be in a relaxed position while urinating.** Relaxing the muscles around the bladder will make it easier to empty the bladder. For women, hovering over the toilet seat may make it hard to relax, so it is best to sit on the toilet seat.
- **Take enough time to fully empty the bladder when urinating.** Rushing may not allow you to do so, and if

urine stays in the bladder too long, it can make a bladder infection more likely.

- **Women should wipe from front to back after using the toilet to prevent gut bacteria from getting into the urethra**. This step is most important after a bowel movement.
- **Urinate after sex**. Sexual activity can move bacteria from the bowel or vaginal cavity to the urethral opening. Both women and men should urinate shortly after sex to lower the risk of infection.
- **Do pelvic floor muscle exercises**. Pelvic floor exercises, also known as "Kegel exercises," help hold urine in the bladder. Daily exercises can strengthen these muscles, which can help keep urine from leaking when you sneeze, cough, lift, laugh, or have a sudden urge to urinate. These exercises also may help avoid infections by strengthening the muscles that help empty the bladder.
- **Wear cotton underwear and loose-fitting clothes**. Wearing loose, cotton clothing will help keep the area around the urethra dry. Tight-fitting pants and nylon underwear can trap moisture and help bacteria grow.
- **Exercise regularly**. Physical activity can help prevent bladder problems and constipation and maintain a healthy weight.
- **Keep a healthy weight**. Overweight people may be at higher risk for leaking urine. Making healthy food choices and being physically active can help maintain a healthy weight.
- **Watch what you eat**. Some people with bladder problems find that certain foods and drinks, such as sodas, artificial sweeteners, spicy foods, citrus fruits and juices, and tomato-based foods, make bladder problems worse. Changing your diet may help you feel better.
- **Drink enough fluids, especially water**. More than half of the human body is made up of water, so it is important that you are drinking enough. How much water you need can vary based on your size, activity level, and where you live. In general, drink enough fluids so that you need to urinate every few hours. Some people need to drink less water because of certain conditions, such as kidney failure

or heart disease. Ask your health-care provider how much fluid is healthy for you.

- **Limit alcohol and caffeine**. For many people, drinking alcohol can make bladder problems worse. Caffeinated drinks (such as coffee, tea, and most sodas) can irritate the bladder and increase symptoms such as frequent or urgent need to urinate. Cutting down may help.
- **Avoid constipation**. Too much stool built up in the colon, called "constipation," can put pressure on the bladder and keep it from expanding as it should. Eating plenty of high-fiber foods such as whole grains, vegetables, and fruits, drinking enough water, and being physically active can help prevent this.
- **Quit smoking**. Bladder problems are more common among people who smoke. Smoking can also increase the risk of bladder cancer. If you smoke, take steps to quit.
- **Know your medications**. Some medications may make it more likely for your bladder to leak urine. Medications that calm your nerves so you can sleep or relax may dull the nerves in the bladder, and you may not feel the urge to go to the bathroom.

COMMON BLADDER PROBLEMS AND WHEN TO SEEK HELP

Bladder problems can disrupt day-to-day life. When people have bladder problems, they may avoid social settings and have a harder time getting tasks done at home or at work. Common bladder problems include urinary tract infections, urinary incontinence, and urinary retention.

Some signs of a bladder problem may include:

- inability to hold urine or leaking urine
- needing to urinate more frequently or urgently
- cloudy urine
- blood in the urine
- pain or burning before, during, or after urinating
- trouble starting or having a weak stream while urinating
- trouble emptying the bladder

If you experience any of these symptoms, talk to your health-care provider.

Treatment for bladder problems may include behavioral and lifestyle changes, exercises, medications, surgery, or a combination of these treatments.[1]

[1] National Institute on Aging (NIA), "15 Tips to Keep Your Bladder Healthy," National Institutes of Health (NIH), January 24, 2022. Available online. URL: www.nia.nih.gov/health/bladder-health-and-incontinence/15-tips-keep-your-bladder-healthy. Accessed October 22, 2024.

Chapter 20 | **Bladder Control Problems (Urinary Incontinence)**

Chapter Contents

Section 20.1 | Understanding Bladder Control Problems

WHAT ARE BLADDER CONTROL PROBLEMS?

Bladder control problems are conditions that affect the way a person holds or releases urine. Accidental loss or leaking of urine, called "urinary incontinence" (UI), is one of the most common bladder control problems. UI is not a disease but a condition that may be related to another health problem or life event, such as prostate problems or pregnancy.

Bladder control problems can be a small annoyance or can greatly affect your quality of life. You may be too embarrassed or afraid to participate in activities because of these problems, or you may be unable to complete your normal routine. For example, you may lose urine while running or coughing, or you may leak urine before you can get to a toilet.

Bladder control problems are common. Proper treatment may improve your quality of life. Talk with a health-care professional about urine leaks. Health-care professionals—especially gynecologists, urologists, and geriatricians—often discuss bladder control problems with patients. Health-care professionals can help treat the problem or manage the symptoms by suggesting simple lifestyle changes. Caregivers may find help from a health-care professional or a support group. The sooner you get help, the sooner UI may improve.

WHAT ARE THE TYPES OF BLADDER CONTROL PROBLEMS?

Types of bladder control problems are identified by their symptoms. The most common bladder control problems include:

- stress incontinence
- urgency incontinence
- reflex incontinence
- overflow incontinence
- functional incontinence
- temporary incontinence
- bedwetting

Stress Incontinence

Stress incontinence occurs when movement—coughing, sneezing, laughing, or physical activity—puts pressure on the bladder and causes urine to leak.

Urgency Incontinence

Urgency incontinence occurs when you have a strong urge or need to urinate, and urine leaks before you can get to a toilet. This type of incontinence is often referred to as "overactive bladder." It happens when certain nerves and bladder muscles do not work together to hold urine in the bladder, and the urine is released at the wrong time.

You can have urgency and stress incontinence at the same time, which is called "mixed incontinence."

Reflex Incontinence

With reflex incontinence, urine leaks without a warning or urge to urinate. This type of incontinence often occurs when your bladder nerves are damaged and do not "talk" to your brain correctly. During reflex incontinence, the bladder contracts at the wrong time, causing urine to leak. Nerve damage from health conditions, such as multiple sclerosis, or from trauma, such as a spinal cord injury, are among the causes of reflex incontinence. Reflex incontinence is sometimes called "unaware" or "unconscious" incontinence.

Overflow Incontinence

Overflow incontinence occurs when the bladder does not empty completely, allowing too much urine to stay in the bladder. As a result, urine leaks because the bladder becomes too full.

Functional Incontinence

Functional incontinence occurs when a physical disability or barrier, or a problem with speaking or thinking, prevents you from reaching the toilet in time. For example, a person in a wheelchair may not be able to get to a toilet in time; someone with arthritis may have trouble unbuttoning their pants; or a person with Alzheimer disease may not realize they need time to get to the toilet.

Temporary Incontinence

Temporary, or transient, incontinence lasts a short time due to a temporary situation, such as using a certain medicine or having an illness that causes leaking. For example, a urinary tract infection (UTI) or a bad cough may cause temporary incontinence.

Bedwetting

Bedwetting, also called "nocturnal enuresis," does not only occur in children. Some adults leak urine while sleeping for a variety of reasons. Certain medications or drinking caffeine or alcohol at night can make it hard to sleep through the night without leaking urine. In some cases, the bladder cannot hold enough urine overnight. Lifestyle changes often can improve these symptoms.

Some people wet the bed because they do not produce enough of a certain hormone at night, which could be a sign of diabetes insipidus. Other health problems, such as a UTI, kidney stones, congestive heart failure, chronic kidney disease, prostate enlargement, or obstructive sleep apnea, can cause bedwetting or frequent urination at night.

HOW COMMON ARE BLADDER CONTROL PROBLEMS?

Bladder control problems are common, especially in women. Researchers estimate that approximately half of all women experience UI. Women are more likely to develop UI during and after pregnancy, childbirth, and menopause. These events and the anatomical structure of the female urinary tract make UI more common in women than in men. Although UI is common, it is not a routine part of being a woman or getting older.

As many as one in three men over the age of 65 may experience accidental urine loss and approximately half of the men who seek treatment for lower urinary tract symptoms experience UI. A man is more likely to develop UI with age because prostate problems occur more frequently with age.

WHO IS MORE LIKELY TO DEVELOP BLADDER CONTROL PROBLEMS?

Factors that make you more likely to develop UI include:

- being female
- being older—as you age, your urinary tract muscles weaken, making it harder to hold in urine
- life events, such as pregnancy, childbirth, and menopause in women and prostate problems in men
- health problems, such as diabetes, obesity, Parkinson disease, multiple sclerosis, or long-lasting constipation
- smoking
- birth defects that involve a problem with the structure of the urinary tract

Your health-care professional can help you find the cause of your bladder control problems and discuss your treatment options.

You are more likely to have a particular type of UI if a family member has that same type of UI. For example, bedwetting often runs in families, and children may outgrow the problem at about the same age their parents did.

WHAT ARE THE COMPLICATIONS OF BLADDER CONTROL PROBLEMS?

Reduced Physical Activity

Physical activity is important for overall health and may prevent further bladder control problems. However, some activities, such as running, jumping, or brisk walking, may cause some people with UI to leak. If you have not found a medicine or other treatment that is right for you, or you want extra peace of mind, new incontinence briefs and pads are discreet and effective at absorbing leaks and controlling odor. New technology and designs can make these products more comfortable to wear and may give you the confidence to get moving again.

Talk with your health-care professional if your bladder control problems are making it difficult for you to be active.

Emotional Distress

Untreated bladder problems can upset your lifestyle. You may avoid activities you once enjoyed. You might stop going to movies, meetings, or events because you do not want to use the restroom in the middle of an activity or have an accident. These lifestyle changes can lead to depression or social anxiety.

If you often feel depressed or anxious about living with bladder control problems, talk with a health-care professional.

Intimacy Problems

Some people may avoid intimacy because they worry they may leak urine during sex. Talk with a health-care professional if your bladder control problems are getting in the way of your sex life. Gynecologists and urologists regularly discuss health problems with patients and can offer solutions.

Related Bladder Symptoms and Problems

If you have UI, you are more likely to have other bladder symptoms or problems, such as:

- urinary frequency
- getting up from sleep to urinate, called "nocturia"
- difficulty urinating
- trouble emptying your bladder fully, called "urinary retention"
- dribbling urine after you think you have finished

When discussing other symptoms of UI, health-care professionals may use the term "LUTS," which stands for lower urinary tract symptoms.

Working with a health-care professional to prevent and treat these related symptoms and problems is important for the health of your bladder and your overall health.[1]

[1] "Definition and Facts for Bladder Control Problems (Urinary Incontinence)," National Institute of Diabetes and Digestive and Kidney Diseases (NIDDK), July 2021. Available online. URL: www.niddk.nih.gov/health-information/urologic-diseases/bladder-control-problems. Accessed October 18, 2024.

Section 20.2 | Identifying and Managing Urinary Incontinence

WHAT ARE BLADDER CONTROL PROBLEMS?

Bladder control problems are conditions that affect the way a person holds or releases urine. Accidental loss or leaking of urine, called "urinary incontinence" (UI), is one of the most common bladder control problems. UI is not a disease but a condition that may be related to another health problem or life event, such as prostate problems or pregnancy.

WHAT ARE THE SYMPTOMS OF BLADDER CONTROL PROBLEMS?

Signs and symptoms of UI can include:

- leaking urine during everyday activities, such as lifting, bending, coughing, or exercising
- being unable to hold in urine after feeling a sudden, strong urge to urinate
- leaking urine without any warning or urge
- being unable to reach a toilet in time
- wetting your bed during sleep
- leaking during sexual activity

WHEN SHOULD I SEE A HEALTH-CARE PROFESSIONAL?

See a health-care professional if you have symptoms of a bladder problem, such as trouble urinating, loss of bladder control, waking to use the bathroom, pelvic pain, or leaking urine.

Bladder problems can affect your quality of life and cause other health issues. Your health-care professional may be able to treat your UI by recommending lifestyle changes or a change in medication.

Seek Care Right Away

See a health-care professional if you:

- cannot pass urine or empty your bladder, which is a sign of urinary retention
- urinate too often—eight or more bathroom visits a day

- see blood in your urine, known as "hematuria"
- have bladder infection symptoms, including painful urination

These symptoms can signal a serious health problem, including inflammation of the bladder, also known as "cystitis," or even bladder cancer.

WHAT CAUSES BLADDER CONTROL PROBLEMS?

Health changes and problems, including those with your nervous system, as well as lifestyle factors, can cause or contribute to UI in women and men.

Health Changes and Problems

Health changes and problems that can lead to UI include:

- aging
- bladder infection
- constipation
- birth defects
- blocked urinary tract—from a tumor or kidney stone
- chronic, or long-lasting, cough
- diabetes
- overweight or obesity
- genitourinary fistulas

Some health problems, such as a urinary tract infection (UTI) or constipation, can be short-term and cause temporary incontinence.

Nerve Damage

Problems with the nervous system are common causes of UI. Nerves carry messages from the bladder to the brain to let it know when the bladder is full. Nerves also carry messages from the brain to the bladder, telling muscles either to tighten or release. The brain decides if it is an acceptable time to urinate. Functional incontinence can occur when there is a problem getting messages from the brain to a part of the urinary tract—usually the bladder, the sphincters, or both.

Bladder nerves and muscles can be damaged or affected by:

- diabetes
- vaginal childbirth
- surgery for prostate cancer
- stroke
- Parkinson disease
- multiple sclerosis
- Alzheimer disease
- brain or spinal cord injury
- anxiety
- heavy metal poisoning

Triggers that may cause a sudden, strong urge to urinate can include drinking or touching water, hearing running water, or being in a cold environment, such as reaching into the freezer at the grocery store.

Lifestyle Factors

Lifestyle factors that make women and men more likely to experience UI include:

- eating habits, such as consuming foods that cause constipation
- drinking habits, such as drinking alcohol or caffeinated or carbonated beverages
- certain medications
- physical inactivity
- smoking

Temporary incontinence is usually a side effect of a medication or a short-term health condition. It can also result from eating and drinking habits, including consuming alcohol or caffeine.[1]

---

[1] "Symptoms and Causes of Bladder Control Problems (Urinary Incontinence)," National Institute of Diabetes and Digestive and Kidney Diseases (NIDDK), July 2021. Available online. URL: www.niddk.nih.gov/health-information/urologic-diseases/bladder-control-problems/symptoms-causes. Accessed October 24, 2024.

CAN I TREAT MY BLADDER CONTROL PROBLEM MYSELF?

Depending on the type of urinary incontinence (UI) you have, your health-care professional may recommend steps you can take to control your symptoms.

Make Lifestyle Changes

You may be able to reduce leaks by making lifestyle changes.

Drink the Right Amount of Liquid at the Right Time

Ask your health-care professional whether you should drink less liquid during the day. However, do not limit liquids to the point of becoming dehydrated. Your health-care professional can tell you how much and when to drink based on your health, activities, and local climate.

To limit nighttime trips to the bathroom, you may want to stop drinking liquids a few hours before bedtime, but only if your health-care professional suggests it. Limiting foods and drinks with caffeine, such as chocolate, tea, coffee, and carbonated beverages, may help reduce leaks. You should also limit alcoholic drinks, which can increase how much urine your body makes.

The amount of urine a person should produce varies between people, depending on how much liquid they drink, sweat, lose by breathing, and take medications.

Be Physically Active

Although you may not feel like being physically active when you have UI, regular physical activity is important for weight management and overall health. Activities such as walking, swimming, biking, and dancing can improve your health. If you are concerned about not having a bathroom nearby during physical activity, find a place with nearby restrooms, such as a shopping mall, community park, or local gym.

Keep a Healthy Weight

Your chances of developing UI and other diseases, such as diabetes, are higher if you are overweight or have obesity. Losing weight can help you have fewer leaks, and avoiding weight gain may prevent

UI. Studies suggest that as your body mass index (BMI) increases, you are more likely to leak. If you are overweight or have obesity, talk with your health-care professional about how to lose weight.

Avoid Constipation

Constipation can worsen urinary tract health and lead to UI. Talk with your health-care professional about drinking more liquids and eating enough fiber to avoid constipation. Health-care professionals use medicines such as anticholinergics, tricyclic antidepressants, and beta-3 agonists to treat UI, but these can cause constipation.

Stop Smoking

If you smoke, seek help to stop. Quitting smoking at any age is beneficial for your bladder health and overall health. Smoking increases your chances of developing stress incontinence because it causes chronic coughing. You might improve your UI if you are able to stop coughing.

Smoking also contributes to most cases of bladder cancer. Some people report that smoking irritates their bladder.

Train Your Bladder

Bladder training involves urinating on a schedule to reduce leaking. Your health-care professional may use your bladder diary to suggest using the bathroom regularly, a method known as "timed voiding." Gradually lengthening the time between trips to the bathroom can help stretch your bladder so it can hold more urine. Record your daily bathroom habits so you and your health-care professional can review your diary.

Do Pelvic Floor Muscle Exercises

Strong pelvic floor muscles hold in urine better than weak muscles. You can strengthen your pelvic floor muscles by doing Kegel exercises. These exercises involve tightening and relaxing the muscles that control urine flow. Researchers have found that women who received pelvic floor muscle training had fewer leaks per day than women who did not receive training. You should not do pelvic floor exercises while urinating.

Men can also benefit from pelvic floor muscle exercises. Strengthening these muscles may help reduce urine leakage, especially dribbling after urination.

A health-care professional, such as a physical therapist trained in pelvic floor therapy, can help you get the most out of your Kegel exercises by improving your core muscle strength. Your core includes your torso muscles, especially the lower back, pelvic floor muscles, and abdomen. These muscles keep your pelvis aligned with your spine, which helps with good posture and balance. Your physical therapist can show you how to perform exercises during daily activities, such as riding in a car or sitting at a desk.

You do not need special equipment for Kegel exercises. However, if you are unsure whether you are doing the exercises correctly, you can learn how to perform Kegel exercises properly by using biofeedback, electrical stimulation, or both. Biofeedback uses special sensors to measure muscle contractions that control urination.

Control Your Urge to Urinate

You may be able to control or suppress the strong urge to urinate, which is called "urge or urgency suppression." With this type of bladder training, you can worry less about finding a bathroom in a hurry. Some people distract themselves to take their minds off needing to urinate. Others find that long, relaxing breaths or holding still can help. Doing pelvic floor exercises to strengthen your pelvic floor may also help control the urge to urinate. Quick, strong squeezes of the pelvic floor muscles can help suppress urgency when it occurs, which may help you reach the toilet before leaking.

HOW CAN I COPE WITH BLADDER CONTROL PROBLEMS?

Protective Products

Even after treatment, you may still leak urine from time to time. Certain products can help you cope with urine leaks:

- **Absorbent, washable incontinence underwear.** Underwear lined with special fabric that absorbs urine.
- **Waterproof underwear.** Protects your clothes from getting wet.

- **Adult incontinence briefs.** Disposable briefs that act like diapers to keep your clothes dry.
- **Pads.** Disposable pads worn in your underwear to absorb leaking urine.
- **Large disposable pads.** Used to protect chairs and beds from urine.
- **Special skin cleaners and creams.** Help keep the skin around the urethra from getting irritated. Creams can help block urine from your skin.
- **Urine deodorizing tablets.** Discuss with your health-care professional whether taking urine deodorizing tablets can make your urine smell less strong.
- **External catheters.** Used by men to collect urine and drain it into a bag attached to the thigh with a strap.

Emotional Support

Bladder control problems are common, yet many people feel too embarrassed to talk about them. At the very least, talk with your health-care professional about your bladder problems. Your health-care professional can help you connect with a support group for people with similar issues.

Consider speaking with your family and friends about your UI. Sharing your struggle may help you manage UI, and you may find that others in your life have similar bladder problems.[2]

Section 20.3 | **Urinary Incontinence in Women**

OVERVIEW OF URINARY INCONTINENCE IN WOMEN

Urinary incontinence is the loss of bladder control or leaking urine. It affects twice as many women as men. This is primarily due to reproductive health events unique to women, such as pregnancy,

[2] "Treatments for Bladder Control Problems (Urinary Incontinence)," National Institute of Diabetes and Digestive and Kidney Diseases (NIDDK), July 2021. Available online. URL: www.niddk.nih.gov/health-information/urologic-diseases/bladder-control-problems/treatment. Accessed October 24, 2024.

childbirth, and menopause, which can affect the bladder, urethra, and other muscles that support these organs.

Urinary incontinence can occur in women at any age, but it is more common in older women. This is likely due to hormonal changes during menopause. More than 4 in 10 women aged 65 and older experience urinary incontinence.

Women undergo unique health events, such as pregnancy, childbirth, and menopause, that may affect the urinary tract and the surrounding muscles. The pelvic floor muscles that support the bladder, urethra, uterus (womb), and bowels may become weaker or damaged. When the muscles supporting the urinary tract are weak, the muscles in the urinary tract must work harder to hold urine until you are ready to urinate. This extra stress or pressure on the bladder and urethra can lead to urinary incontinence or leakage.

Additionally, the female urethra is shorter than the male urethra. Any weakness or damage to the urethra in a woman is more likely to result in urinary incontinence because there is less muscle keeping the urine in until you are ready to urinate.

TYPES OF URINARY INCONTINENCE IN WOMEN

The two most common types of urinary incontinence in women are:

- **Stress incontinence**. This is the most common type of incontinence, particularly affecting younger women. Stress incontinence occurs when there is stress or pressure on the bladder. It can happen when weak pelvic floor muscles put pressure on the bladder and urethra, making them work harder. Everyday actions that utilize the pelvic floor muscles, such as coughing, sneezing, or laughing, can cause urine leakage. Sudden movements and physical activity can also lead to leakage.
- **Urge incontinence**. With urge incontinence, urine leakage usually occurs after a strong, sudden urge to urinate and before you can reach a bathroom. Some women with urge incontinence can get to a bathroom in time but feel the urge to urinate more than eight

times a day and may not urinate much once they arrive. Urge incontinence is sometimes referred to as "overactive bladder" and is more common in older women. It can occur unexpectedly, such as during sleep, after drinking water, or when hearing or touching running water.

Many women experience both stress and urge incontinence, which is referred to as "mixed incontinence."

FACTORS CONTRIBUTING TO URINARY INCONTINENCE IN WOMEN

Pregnancy

As many as 4 in 10 women experience urinary incontinence during pregnancy. During this time, as the unborn baby grows, it exerts pressure on the bladder, urethra, and pelvic floor muscles. Over time, this pressure may weaken the pelvic floor muscles and lead to leaks or difficulties passing urine.

Most bladder control issues during pregnancy resolve after childbirth when the muscles have time to heal. If you are still experiencing bladder problems six weeks after childbirth, consult your doctor, nurse, or midwife.

Problems during labor and childbirth, especially with vaginal delivery, can weaken pelvic floor muscles and damage the nerves that control the bladder. Most bladder control problems that arise from labor and delivery improve after the muscles have healed. If you continue to have bladder issues six weeks after childbirth, speak with your health-care provider.

Hormonal Changes and Aging

Some women experience bladder control problems after they stop having periods. Researchers believe that low levels of the hormone estrogen after menopause may weaken the urethra, which helps keep urine in the bladder until you are ready to urinate.

Additionally, like all muscles, the bladder and urethra muscles lose some strength as you age. This means you may not be able to hold as much urine as you get older.

RISK REDUCTION STRATEGIES FOR URINARY INCONTINENCE

Although you cannot always prevent urinary incontinence, you can take steps to lower your risk:

- Practice Kegel exercises daily, especially during pregnancy, after consulting your doctor, nurse, or midwife.
- Maintain a healthy weight.
- Eat fiber-rich foods to help prevent constipation.[1]

Section 20.4 | Urinary Incontinence in Children

Children may have a bladder control problem—also called "urinary incontinence" (UI)—if they leak urine by accident and are past the age of toilet training. They may not stay dry during the day, which is referred to as "daytime wetting," or at night, which is known as "bedwetting."

Children typically gain control over their bladders between ages two and four—each at their own pace. Occasional wetting is common even in four- to six-year-old children.

By age four, when most children stay dry during the day, daytime wetting can be very upsetting and embarrassing. By ages five or six, children may have a bedwetting problem if the bed is wet once or twice a week over a few months.

Most bladder control problems disappear naturally as children grow older. When needed, a health-care professional can check for conditions that may lead to wetting.

Loss of urine is almost never due to laziness, a strong will, emotional problems, or poor toilet training. Parents and caregivers should always approach this problem with understanding and patience.

[1] Office on Women's Health (OWH), "Urinary Incontinence," U.S. Department of Health and Human Services (HHS), February 22, 2021. Available online. URL: www.womenshealth.gov/a-z-topics/urinary-incontinence. Accessed October 17, 2024.

WHAT ARE THE TYPES OF BLADDER CONTROL PROBLEMS IN CHILDREN?

Children usually experience one of two main bladder control problems:

- daytime wetting, also called "diurnal enuresis"
- bedwetting, also called "nocturnal enuresis"

Some children may have trouble controlling their bladders both day and night.

Daytime Wetting

For infants and toddlers, wetting is a normal part of development. Children gradually learn to control their bladders as they grow older. Problems that can occur during this process and lead to daytime wetting include:

- **Holding urine too long.** Your child's bladder can overfill and leak urine.
- **Overactive bladder.** Your child's bladder squeezes without warning, causing frequent trips to the toilet and wet clothes.
- **Underactive bladder.** Your child uses the toilet only a few times a day, with little urge to do so. Children may have a weak or interrupted stream of urine.
- **Disordered urination.** Your child's bladder muscles and nerves do not work together smoothly. Certain muscles may cut off urine flow too soon, leading to leakage of urine left in the bladder.

Bedwetting

Children who wet the bed fall into two groups: those who have never been dry at night and those who started wetting the bed again after staying dry for six months.

WHO IS MORE LIKELY TO HAVE BLADDER CONTROL PROBLEMS?

Daytime wetting is more common in girls than boys.

Bedwetting is more common in boys and in all children whose parents wet the bed when they were young. Your child's chances of wetting the bed are about one in three when one parent was affected as a child. If both parents were affected, the chances that your child will wet the bed are 7 in 10.

Most children with bladder control problems are physically and emotionally normal. Certain health conditions can make a child more likely to experience wetting, including:

- a bladder or kidney infection (urinary tract infection)
- constipation—fewer than two bowel movements a week, or painful or hard-to-pass stool
- nerve problems, such as those seen with spina bifida, a birth defect
- vesicoureteral reflux (VUR), or backward flow of urine from the bladder to the kidneys
- diabetes, a condition in which blood glucose, also called "blood sugar," is too high
- problems with the structure of the urinary tract, such as a blockage or a narrowed urethra
- obstructive sleep apnea (OSA), a condition in which breathing is interrupted during sleep, often due to inflamed or enlarged tonsils
- attention deficit hyperactivity disorder (ADHD)

WHAT ARE THE COMPLICATIONS OF BLADDER CONTROL PROBLEMS?

Children can manage or outgrow most bladder control problems with no lasting health effects. However, accidental wetting can cause emotional distress and poor self-esteem for a child, as well as frustration for families.

Bladder control problems can sometimes lead to bladder or kidney infections (UTIs). Bedwetting that is never treated during childhood can persist into the teen years and adulthood, causing emotional distress.

WHEN SHOULD MY CHILD SEE A DOCTOR ABOUT BLADDER CONTROL PROBLEMS?

If you or your child are worried about accidental wetting, talk with a health-care professional. They can check for medical problems and offer treatment or reassure you that your child is developing normally.

Take your child to a health-care professional if there are signs of a medical problem:

- Symptoms of a bladder infection, such as:
  - pain or burning when urinating
  - cloudy, dark, bloody, or foul-smelling urine
  - urinating more often than usual
  - strong urges to urinate but passing only a small amount of urine
  - pain in the lower belly area or back
  - crying while urinating
  - fever
  - restlessness
- Your child dribbles urine or has a weak urine stream, which can indicate a birth defect in the urinary tract
- Your child was dry but started wetting again

Although each child is unique, providers often use a child's age to decide when to look for a bladder control problem. In general:

- by age four, most children are dry during the day
- by ages five or six, most children are dry at night

HOW CAN I HELP MY CHILD COPE WITH BLADDER CONTROL PROBLEMS?

Your patience, understanding, and encouragement are vital to helping your child cope with a bladder control problem. If you think a health problem may be causing your child's wetting, make an appointment with your child's health-care provider.

Clothing, Bedding, and Wearable Products

For children with daytime wetting, clothes that come on and off easily may help prevent accidents. A wristwatch alarm set to vibrate can privately remind your child to visit the restroom without help from a teacher or parent.

For children who wet the bed, the following practices can make life easier and may boost your child's confidence:

- Leave out dry pajamas and towels so your child can clean up easily.
- Layer waterproof pads and fitted sheets on the bed. Your child can quickly pull off wet bedding and place it in a hamper. Fewer signs of wetting may help your child feel less embarrassed.
- Have your child help with the cleanup and laundry the next day, but do not make it a punishment.
- Ensure your child showers or bathes daily to wash away the smell of urine.
- Plan to stop using diapers, training pants, or disposable training pants, except when sleeping away from home. These items may discourage your child from getting out of bed to use the restroom.

HOW CAN I HELP MY CHILD PREVENT BLADDER CONTROL PROBLEMS?

While you cannot always prevent a bladder control problem, especially bedwetting, which is a common pattern of normal child development, good habits may help your child have more dry days and nights, including:

- Avoid or treat constipation.
- Urinate every two to three hours during the day—four to seven times total in a day.
- Drink the right amount of liquid, with most liquids consumed between morning and about 5 p.m. Ask your child's health-care provider how much liquid is healthy based on age, weather, and activities.

- Avoid drinks with caffeine or bubbles, citrus juices, and sports drinks, as these may irritate the bladder or produce extra urine.[1]

Section 20.5 | Urinary Incontinence in Older Adults

URINARY INCONTINENCE AND ITS CAUSES

Urinary incontinence refers to the "accidental leakage of urine." While it can happen to anyone, urinary incontinence, also known as "overactive bladder," is more common in older individuals, especially women. Bladder control issues can be embarrassing and may lead people to avoid their normal activities. However, incontinence can often be stopped or controlled.

Located in the lower abdomen, the bladder is a hollow organ that is part of the urinary system, which also includes the kidneys, ureters, and urethra. During urination, muscles in the bladder tighten to move urine into the tube-shaped urethra. Simultaneously, the muscles around the urethra relax, allowing urine to pass out of the body. When the muscles in and around the bladder do not function properly, urine can leak, resulting in urinary incontinence.

Incontinence can occur for many reasons, including urinary tract infections (UTIs), vaginal infections or irritation, or constipation. Some medications can cause temporary bladder control problems. When incontinence persists, it may be due to:

- weak bladder or pelvic floor muscles
- overactive bladder muscles
- damage to nerves that control the bladder from diseases such as multiple sclerosis, diabetes, or Parkinson disease
- diseases such as arthritis that may make it difficult to reach the bathroom in time

[1] "Bladder Control Problems and Bedwetting in Children," National Institute of Diabetes and Digestive and Kidney Diseases (NIDDK), September 2017. Available online. URL: www.niddk.nih.gov/health-information/urologic-diseases/bladder-control-problems-bedwetting-children. Accessed October 18, 2024.

- pelvic organ prolapse, which occurs when pelvic organs (such as the bladder, rectum, or uterus) shift out of their normal position into the vagina or anus. When pelvic organs are displaced, the bladder and urethra may not function normally, leading to urine leakage

Most incontinence in men is related to the prostate gland. Male incontinence may be caused by:

- prostatitis, a painful inflammation of the prostate gland
- injury or damage to nerves or muscles from surgery
- an enlarged prostate gland, which can lead to benign prostatic hyperplasia, a condition in which the prostate grows as men age

TYPES OF URINARY INCONTINENCE

There are several types of incontinence:

- **Stress incontinence**. This occurs when urine leaks due to pressure on the bladder, such as during exercise, coughing, sneezing, laughing, or lifting heavy objects. It is the most common type of bladder control problem in younger and middle-aged women and may begin later, around the time of menopause.
- **Urge incontinence**. This happens when individuals experience a sudden need to urinate and cannot hold their urine long enough to reach the toilet. It may be a problem for people with diabetes, Alzheimer disease, Parkinson disease, multiple sclerosis, or those who have had a stroke.
- **Overflow incontinence**. This occurs when small amounts of urine leak from a bladder that is always full. A man may have difficulty emptying his bladder if an enlarged prostate is blocking the urethra. Diabetes and spinal cord injuries can also lead to this type of incontinence.
- **Functional incontinence**. This occurs in many older individuals who have normal bladder control but face barriers to reaching the toilet due to conditions such as arthritis.

TREATING AND MANAGING URINARY INCONTINENCE

Today, there are more treatments and ways to manage urinary incontinence than ever before. The choice of treatment depends on the type of bladder control problem you have, its severity, and what best fits your lifestyle. Generally, the simplest and safest treatments should be tried first.

A combination of treatments may help improve bladder control. Your doctor may suggest the following:

Bladder Control Training

- **Pelvic muscle exercises**. Also known as "Kegel exercises," these strengthen the muscles that support the bladder, helping you hold urine and avoid leaks.
- **Urgency suppression**. This technique helps control strong urges to urinate, allowing you to reach a toilet in time. Techniques include distraction, deep breathing, holding still, and squeezing the pelvic floor muscles.
- **Timed voiding**. This involves scheduling regular trips to the toilet and gradually extending the time between visits to train your bladder.

Medical Treatments

Medications that come in pill, liquid, or patch form may be prescribed to help with bladder control problems. However, some medications for overactive bladder have been associated with a higher risk of cognitive decline in adults over age 65. Discuss with your doctor which medications, if any, would work best for you.

- **Vaginal estrogen cream**. This may help relieve urge or stress incontinence by applying a low dose of estrogen cream directly to the vaginal walls and urethral tissue.
- **Bulking agents**. These can help close the bladder opening. Doctors can inject a bulking gel or paste that thickens the area around the urethra, which may reduce stress incontinence but may need to be repeated.
- **Medical devices**. These may include catheters to drain urine from the bladder, urethral inserts to prevent

leakage, and vaginal pessary rings to provide pressure to lessen leakage.
- **Biofeedback.** This uses sensors to help you become aware of signals from your body, aiding in regaining control over the muscles in your bladder and urethra.
- **Electrical nerve stimulation.** This sends mild electric currents to the nerves around the bladder that help control urination and the bladder's reflexes.
- **Surgery.** This can sometimes improve or cure incontinence if caused by a change in the position of the bladder or blockage due to an enlarged prostate.

Behavioral and Lifestyle Changes

Changing your lifestyle may help with bladder problems. Losing weight, quitting smoking, avoiding alcohol, choosing water instead of other drinks, and limiting fluid intake before bedtime can help manage some bladder issues. Preventing constipation and avoiding heavy lifting may also contribute to reducing incontinence. Even after treatment, some individuals may still experience occasional leaks. Various bladder control products, such as disposable briefs or underwear, furniture pads, and urine deodorizing pills, can assist in managing symptoms.

Managing Incontinence in People with Alzheimer Disease

People in the later stages of Alzheimer disease often experience urinary incontinence. This can result from not realizing they need to urinate, forgetting to go to the bathroom, or being unable to find the toilet. To help manage this issue:
- Avoid drinks such as caffeinated coffee, tea, and sodas, which may increase urination, but do not limit water intake.
- Keep hallways clear and the bathroom clutter-free, with a light on at all times.
- Provide regular bathroom breaks.
- Use underwear that is easy to put on and take off, along with absorbent briefs or underwear for trips away from home.

WHEN TO SEE A HEALTH-CARE PROVIDER AND WHAT TO EXPECT

Talk to your health-care provider if you experience urinary incontinence or any signs of a bladder problem, such as:

- needing to urinate more frequently or suddenly
- cloudy urine
- blood in the urine
- pain while urinating
- urinating eight or more times in one day
- passing only small amounts of urine after experiencing strong urges to urinate
- trouble starting or having a weak urine stream while urinating[1]

[1] National Institute on Aging (NIA), "Urinary Incontinence in Older Adults," National Institutes of Health (NIH), January 24, 2022. Available online. URL: www.nia.nih.gov/health/urinary-incontinence-older-adults. Accessed October 18, 2024.

Chapter 21 | Prostate Problems

Chapter Contents

WHAT IS THE PROSTATE?

The prostate is a walnut-shaped gland that is part of a man's reproductive system, which also includes the penis, scrotum, and testicles. The prostate produces fluid that is included in semen, which is a mix of sperm and prostate fluid. Prostate fluid is essential for a man's ability to father children.

The prostate is located in front of the rectum and just below the bladder. The gland surrounds the urethra at the neck of the bladder, which is the area where the urethra joins the bladder. The urethra is the tube that carries urine from the bladder to the outside of the body. In men, the urethra also carries semen out through the penis during sexual climax, or ejaculation. The bladder and urethra are parts of the lower urinary tract.

Both urine and semen pass through the urethra, traversing the prostate.

WHAT CAUSES PROSTATE PROBLEMS?

The causes of prostate problems may include:

- prostatitis
- benign prostatic hyperplasia (BPH)

Your doctor may not always know the exact cause of your prostate problem.

Prostatitis

The cause of prostatitis depends on whether you have chronic prostatitis or bacterial prostatitis.

- **Chronic prostatitis**. The exact cause of chronic prostatitis is unknown. Researchers believe that an infection by tiny organisms, though not bacteria, may cause chronic prostatitis. Other potential causes include chemicals in your urine, your body's response to a previous urinary tract infection (UTI), or nerve damage in your pelvic area. Most of the time, doctors do not find any infection in men with chronic prostatitis.

- **Bacterial prostatitis.** Bacterial prostatitis is caused by bacteria, which are tiny organisms that can lead to infection.

Benign Prostatic Hyperplasia

Doctors do not know the exact cause of BPH. Changes in male hormone levels in older men, aging, inflammation, and fibrosis may play a role in the development of BPH. "Fibrosis" refers to the formation of excess tissue around your organs, which can become thick and stiff.

WHO DEVELOPS PROSTATE PROBLEMS AND HOW COMMON ARE THEY?

Any man can develop a prostate problem. Prostatitis can affect men of all ages, but it is the most common prostate issue in men younger than age 50. BPH is the most common prostate problem in men older than age 50.

- **Prostatitis.** If you have a UTI, you may be more likely to develop bacterial prostatitis. If you have nerve damage in your lower urinary tract or experience emotional stress, you may be more susceptible to chronic prostatitis.
- **BPH.** Men younger than age 40 rarely experience BPH symptoms. The prevalence of BPH symptoms increases with age. If you have a family history of BPH, you may be more likely to develop it. Other factors that increase your risk for BPH may include certain medical conditions and lifestyle choices.

WHAT ARE THE SYMPTOMS OF PROSTATE PROBLEMS?

The symptoms of a prostate problem may include issues with urination and bladder control, which involves the ability to delay, start, or stop urination. These problems can lead to:

- frequent trips to the bathroom
- a sudden need to rush to the bathroom, often resulting in difficulty urinating or only passing a small amount

- leakage or dribbling of urine
- a weak urine stream

Depending on the cause of your prostate problems, you may experience additional symptoms.

Prostatitis

If you have chronic prostatitis, your symptoms may include long-lasting pain and discomfort in:

- the penis or scrotum
- the area between your scrotum and anus
- the belly
- the lower back

If you have bacterial prostatitis, your symptoms may come on suddenly or develop slowly over time. You may have difficulty completely emptying your bladder and may experience fever, chills, or body aches.

Benign Prostatic Hyperplasia

If you have BPH, you may need to wake up frequently to urinate during the night. Your urine may have an unusual color or smell, and you may experience pain while urinating or after ejaculation.

HOW DOES MY DOCTOR KNOW IF I HAVE A PROSTATE PROBLEM?

Your doctor can diagnose a prostate problem based on:

- your medical and family history
- a physical exam, including a digital rectal exam of your prostate
- tests on your urine, blood, and lower urinary tract
- ultrasound
- prostate biopsy

HOW CAN I PREVENT A PROSTATE PROBLEM?

Researchers have not identified specific ways to prevent prostate problems. Men with a higher risk of developing prostate problems should discuss any lower urinary tract symptoms with their doctor and consider regular prostate exams. Recognizing lower urinary tract symptoms and understanding whether you have a prostate problem can facilitate early treatment and reduce the effect of prostate issues.[1]

Section 21.2 | **Prostatitis**

WHAT IS PROSTATITIS?

Prostatitis is a frequently painful condition that involves inflammation of the prostate and sometimes the areas around the prostate.

Scientists have identified four types of prostatitis:

- chronic prostatitis or chronic pelvic pain syndrome
- acute bacterial prostatitis
- chronic bacterial prostatitis
- asymptomatic inflammatory prostatitis

Men with asymptomatic inflammatory prostatitis do not have symptoms. A health-care provider may diagnose asymptomatic inflammatory prostatitis when testing for other urinary tract or reproductive tract disorders. This type of prostatitis does not cause complications and does not require treatment.

HOW COMMON IS PROSTATITIS?

Prostatitis is the most common urinary tract problem for men younger than 50 and the third most common for men older than 50. It accounts for about 2 million visits to health-care providers in the United States each year.

[1] "Prostate Problems," National Institute of Diabetes and Digestive and Kidney Diseases (NIDDK), March 2016. Available online. URL: www.niddk.nih.gov/health-information/urologic-diseases/prostate-problems. Accessed October 18, 2024.

Chronic prostatitis or chronic pelvic pain syndrome is characterized by several aspects:

- It is the most common and least understood form of prostatitis.
- It can occur in men of any age group.
- It affects 10–15 percent of the U.S. male population.

WHO IS MORE LIKELY TO DEVELOP PROSTATITIS?

The factors that affect a man's chances of developing prostatitis differ depending on the type.

Chronic Prostatitis/Chronic Pelvic Pain Syndrome

Men with nerve damage in the lower urinary tract due to surgery or trauma may be more likely to develop chronic prostatitis/chronic pelvic pain syndrome. Psychological stress may also increase a man's chances of developing the condition.

Acute and Chronic Bacterial Prostatitis

Men with lower UTIs may be more likely to develop bacterial prostatitis. Recurring or difficult-to-treat UTIs may lead to chronic bacterial prostatitis.

WHAT CAUSES PROSTATITIS?

The causes of prostatitis differ depending on the type.

Chronic Prostatitis or Chronic Pelvic Pain Syndrome

The exact cause of chronic prostatitis/chronic pelvic pain syndrome is unknown. Researchers believe a microorganism, though not a bacterial infection, may cause the condition. This type of prostatitis may relate to chemicals in the urine, the immune system's response to a previous urinary tract infection (UTI), or nerve damage in the pelvic area.

Acute and Chronic Bacterial Prostatitis

A bacterial infection of the prostate causes bacterial prostatitis. The acute type happens suddenly and lasts a short time, while the chronic type develops slowly and lasts a long time, often years. The infection may occur when bacteria travel from the urethra into the prostate.

WHAT ARE THE SYMPTOMS OF PROSTATITIS?

Each type of prostatitis has a range of symptoms that vary depending on the cause and may not be the same for every man. Many symptoms are similar to those of other conditions.

Chronic Prostatitis/Chronic Pelvic Pain Syndrome

The main symptoms can include pain or discomfort lasting three or more months in one or more of the following areas:

- between the scrotum and anus
- the central lower abdomen
- the penis
- the scrotum
- the lower back

Pain during or after ejaculation is another common symptom. A man with chronic prostatitis/chronic pelvic pain syndrome may experience pain spread out around the pelvic area or may have pain in one or more areas at the same time. The pain may come and go and appear suddenly or gradually. Other symptoms may include:

- pain in the urethra during or after urination
- pain in the penis during or after urination
- urinary frequency—urination eight or more times a day, as the bladder begins to contract even when it contains small amounts of urine, causing more frequent urination
- urinary urgency—the inability to delay urination
- a weak or interrupted urine stream

Acute Bacterial Prostatitis

The symptoms of acute bacterial prostatitis come on suddenly and are severe. Men should seek immediate medical care. Symptoms may include:

- urinary frequency
- urinary urgency

- fever
- chills
- a burning feeling or pain during urination
- pain in the genital area, groin, lower abdomen, or lower back
- nocturia—frequent urination during periods of sleep
- nausea and vomiting
- body aches
- urinary retention—the inability to empty the bladder completely
- trouble starting a urine stream
- a weak or interrupted urine stream
- urinary blockage—the complete inability to urinate
- a UTI, as indicated by bacteria and infection-fighting cells in the urine

Chronic Bacterial Prostatitis

The symptoms of chronic bacterial prostatitis are similar to those of acute bacterial prostatitis, although not as severe. This type of prostatitis often develops slowly and can last three or more months. The symptoms may come and go, or they may be mild all the time. Chronic bacterial prostatitis may occur after previous treatment of acute bacterial prostatitis or a UTI. Symptoms may include:

- urinary frequency
- urinary urgency
- a burning feeling or pain during urination
- pain in the genital area, groin, lower abdomen, or lower back
- nocturia
- painful ejaculation
- urinary retention
- trouble starting a urine stream
- a weak or interrupted urine stream
- urinary blockage
- a UTI

HOW IS PROSTATITIS DIAGNOSED?

A health-care provider diagnoses prostatitis based on:

- a personal and family medical history
- a physical exam
- medical tests

A health-care provider may have to rule out other conditions that cause similar signs and symptoms before diagnosing prostatitis.

HOW IS PROSTATITIS TREATED?

Treatment depends on the type of prostatitis.

Chronic Prostatitis/Chronic Pelvic Pain Syndrome

Treatment for chronic prostatitis/chronic pelvic pain syndrome aims to decrease pain, discomfort, and inflammation. A wide range of symptoms exists, and no single treatment works for every man. Although antibiotics will not help treat nonbacterial prostatitis, a urologist may prescribe them, at least initially, until the urologist can rule out a bacterial infection. A urologist may prescribe other medications, including:

- silodosin (Rapaflo)
- 5-alpha reductase inhibitors such as finasteride (Proscar) and dutasteride (Avodart)
- nonsteroidal anti-inflammatory drugs (NSAIDs) such as aspirin, ibuprofen, and naproxen sodium
- glycosaminoglycans such as chondroitin sulfate
- muscle relaxants such as cyclobenzaprine (Amrix, Flexeril) and clonazepam (Klonopin)
- neuromodulators such as amitriptyline, nortriptyline (Aventyl, Pamelor), and pregabalin (Lyrica)

Alternative treatments may include:

- warm baths, called "sitz baths"
- local heat therapy with hot water bottles or heating pads

- physical therapy, such as:
  - Kegel exercises—tightening and relaxing the muscles that hold urine in the bladder and hold the bladder in its proper position. also called "pelvic muscle exercises"
  - myofascial release—pressing and stretching, sometimes with cooling and warming, of the muscles and soft tissues in the lower back, pelvic region, and upper legs. Also known as "myofascial trigger point release"
  - relaxation exercises
  - biofeedback
- phytotherapy with plant extracts such as quercetin, bee pollen, and saw palmetto
- acupuncture

Acute Bacterial Prostatitis

A urologist treats acute bacterial prostatitis with antibiotics. The antibiotic prescribed may depend on the type of bacteria causing the infection. Urologists usually prescribe oral antibiotics for at least two weeks. The infection may come back; therefore, some urologists recommend taking oral antibiotics for six to eight weeks. Severe cases of acute prostatitis may require a short hospital stay so men can receive fluids and antibiotics through an intravenous (IV) tube. After the IV treatment, the man will need to take oral antibiotics for two to four weeks. Most cases of acute bacterial prostatitis clear up completely with medication and slight changes to diet. The urologist may recommend:

- avoiding or reducing the intake of substances that irritate the bladder, such as alcohol, caffeinated beverages, and acidic and spicy foods
- increasing the intake of liquids, 64–128 ounces per day, to urinate often and help flush bacteria from the bladder

Chronic Bacterial Prostatitis

A urologist treats chronic bacterial prostatitis with antibiotics; however, treatment requires a longer course of therapy. The urologist may prescribe a low dose of antibiotics for up to six months to prevent recurrent infection. The urologist may also prescribe a different antibiotic or use a combination of antibiotics if the infection keeps returning. The urologist may recommend increasing the intake of liquids and avoiding or reducing the intake of substances that irritate the bladder.

A urologist may use alpha-blockers that treat chronic prostatitis/chronic pelvic pain syndrome to treat urinary retention caused by chronic bacterial prostatitis. These medications help relax the bladder muscles near the prostate and lessen symptoms such as painful urination. Men may require surgery to treat urinary retention caused by chronic bacterial prostatitis. Surgically removing scar tissue in the urethra often improves urine flow and reduces urinary retention.[1]

Section 21.3 | **Benign Prostatic Hyperplasia**

Benign prostatic hyperplasia (BPH) is a condition in which the prostate gland grows larger than normal, but this growth is not caused by cancer.

The prostate has two main growth phases. The first occurs early in puberty when the prostate doubles in size. The second begins around age 25 and continues throughout life. BPH often develops late in the second growth phase.

WHO IS MORE LIKELY TO HAVE BENIGN PROSTATIC HYPERPLASIA?

You are more likely to develop BPH if you:

- are 40 or older
- have a family history of BPH
- have certain medical conditions, such as heart and blood vessel disease, type 2 diabetes, obesity, chronic kidney disease, or erectile dysfunction (ED)
- are not physically active

[1] "Prostatitis: Inflammation of the Prostate," National Institute of Diabetes and Digestive and Kidney Diseases (NIDDK), July 2014. Available online. URL: www.niddk.nih.gov/health-information/urologic-diseases/prostate-problems/prostatitis-inflammation-prostate. Accessed October 24, 2024.

WHAT ARE THE COMPLICATIONS OF BENIGN PROSTATIC HYPERPLASIA?

An enlarged prostate can cause problems with bladder emptying. As the prostate grows, it squeezes the urethra. Consequently, the bladder muscles have to work harder to push urine through the narrowed urethra, which may worsen urinary symptoms. Eventually, the bladder muscles may weaken and become unable to empty completely, leaving some urine in the bladder. This condition is known as "urinary retention."

Other complications can include:

- blood in your urine, called "hematuria"
- urinary tract infections (UTIs)
- kidney disease
- bladder stones

WHAT ARE THE SYMPTOMS OF BENIGN PROSTATIC HYPERPLASIA?

If you have BPH, you may experience:

- difficulty starting a urine stream or emptying your bladder
- a weak or interrupted urine stream, or dribbling at the end of urination
- nocturia (waking up at night to urinate)
- urinary urgency (a sudden need to urinate)
- increased urinary frequency
- pain during urination

HOW DO HEALTH-CARE PROFESSIONALS DIAGNOSE BENIGN PROSTATIC HYPERPLASIA?

A health-care provider diagnoses benign prostatic hyperplasia based on:

- a personal and family medical history
- a physical exam
- medical tests

HOW DO HEALTH-CARE PROFESSIONALS TREAT BENIGN PROSTATIC HYPERPLASIA?

Benign prostatic hyperplasia can be treated with watchful waiting, medications, or surgery. A health-care professional will consider the severity of your symptoms and how they affect your quality of life before discussing treatment options with you.

CAN I PREVENT BENIGN PROSTATIC HYPERPLASIA?

Researchers have not identified a way to prevent BPH, but being physically active may help reduce your risk. If you have risk factors for BPH, talk with a health-care professional about any lower urinary tract symptoms you have and how often you may need a prostate exam. Early treatment can help minimize the effects of BPH on your quality of life.[1]

[1] "Enlarged Prostate (Benign Prostatic Hyperplasia)," National Institute of Diabetes and Digestive and Kidney Diseases (NIDDK), June 2024. Available online. URL: www.niddk.nih.gov/health-information/urologic-diseases/prostate-problems/prostate-enlargement-benign-prostatic-hyperplasia. Accessed October 18, 2024.

Chapter 22 | Urinary Retention

WHAT IS URINARY RETENTION?

Urinary retention is a condition in which you are unable to empty all the urine from your bladder. It is not a disease but rather a condition that may be related to other health problems, such as prostate issues in men or a cystocele in women. Urinary retention can be classified as acute—sudden inability to urinate at all—or chronic—gradual inability to empty the bladder.

Acute Urinary Retention

Acute urinary retention occurs suddenly and lasts only a short time. Individuals with acute urinary retention are unable to urinate, even though they have a full bladder.

Acute urinary retention can cause severe pain and may be life-threatening. If you are suddenly unable to urinate, it is important to seek emergency medical treatment immediately.

Chronic Urinary Retention

Chronic urinary retention develops over time. Individuals with chronic urinary retention can urinate but cannot completely empty the urine from their bladders. Many people with chronic urinary retention are unaware of their condition because they may not experience any noticeable symptoms.

WHO IS MORE LIKELY TO DEVELOP URINARY RETENTION?

Urinary retention affects both men and women, but it is more common in men, particularly as they age. Men who have benign prostatic hyperplasia (BPH)—a condition in which the prostate gland is enlarged—are more likely to develop urinary retention. As the prostate enlarges, it pushes against the urethra, blocking the flow of urine from the bladder. BPH is a common prostate problem for men older than 50.

WHAT ARE THE SYMPTOMS OF URINARY RETENTION?

Acute Urinary Retention

Symptoms of acute urinary retention may include:

- inability to urinate
- severe pain in the lower abdomen
- an urgent need to urinate
- swelling of the lower abdomen

Chronic Urinary Retention

Chronic urinary retention develops over time and may cause few or no symptoms, making it difficult to detect. If chronic urinary retention does cause symptoms, they may include:

- inability to completely empty your bladder when urinating
- frequent urination in small amounts
- difficulty starting the flow of urine, known as "hesitancy"
- a slow urine stream
- an urgent need to urinate, but with little success
- feeling the need to urinate after finishing urination
- leaking urine without any warning or urge
- lower abdominal pain or discomfort

WHAT CAUSES URINARY RETENTION?

The causes of urinary retention are related to either a blockage that partially or fully prevents urine from leaving your bladder or urethra, or your bladder not being able to generate sufficient force to expel all the urine.

HOW DO HEALTH-CARE PROFESSIONALS DIAGNOSE URINARY RETENTION?

Health-care professionals diagnose urinary retention using your medical history, a physical exam, and a post-void residual urine measurement. Your health-care professional may also order lab and other diagnostic tests to help determine the cause of your urinary retention.

HOW DO HEALTH-CARE PROFESSIONALS TREAT URINARY RETENTION?

Treatment for urinary retention depends on whether it is acute or chronic and on the underlying cause.

Draining the Bladder

For acute urinary retention, a health-care professional will immediately drain the urine from your bladder using a catheter. This procedure alleviates pain and helps prevent damage to the bladder and kidneys.

If you have chronic urinary retention, your health-care professional will first attempt to diagnose and treat the underlying cause. However, if the retention persists or becomes severe, your health-care professional may need to use a catheter to drain urine from your bladder.

In some cases, individuals with urinary retention may need to continue using a catheter to drain urine until the issue can be resolved. The catheter can be either indwelling (left in the bladder for a short or long period) or intermittent (inserted to drain the bladder as needed and then removed). If you need to use an intermittent catheter, a health-care professional can teach you how to use it.

Medicines

Your health-care professional may recommend medications to help treat the medical condition causing your urinary retention:

- 5-alpha reductase inhibitors help stop the growth of or shrink the prostate, improving urine flow. Examples include dutasteride and finasteride.
- Alpha-blockers alleviate the symptoms of prostate enlargement (BPH) by relaxing muscles in the bladder neck and prostate, making it easier to urinate. Examples include alfuzosin, doxazosin, prazosin, silodosin, tadalafil, tamsulosin, and terazosin.

- A combination of a 5-alpha-reductase inhibitor and an alpha-blocker, such as finasteride and doxazosin or dutasteride and tamsulosin, may be more effective than an individual medication.
- Antibiotics treat infections that may cause urinary retention, such as UTIs and prostatitis.

In some cases, certain medications may contribute to urinary retention. If your health-care professional suspects that a medication is causing your retention, you may be advised to lower the dose or discontinue its use.

All medications, including over-the-counter ones, can have side effects. Always consult your health-care professional before using any medication for more than a few days.

Medical Procedures and Devices

Your health-care professional may recommend medical procedures or devices to treat your urinary retention, depending on the underlying cause. Examples include:

- **Cystoscopy**. Using a cystoscope to examine the urethra and bladder for blockages, such as urinary tract stones.
- **Laser therapy**. This technique employs a strong beam of light to treat enlarged prostate tissue by breaking up the blockage and reducing obstruction.
- **Prostatic urethral lift (UroLift)**. Tiny implants lift and hold the prostate away from the urethra, allowing urine to flow more freely.
- **Transurethral electrovaporization**. This procedure uses heat to vaporize enlarged prostate tissue.
- **Transurethral water vapor therapy (Rezum)**. This therapy uses water vapor, or steam, to shrink an enlarged prostate.
- **Urethral dilation**. Gradually increasing the size of the urethral opening by stretching scar tissue to treat urethral strictures.
- **Vaginal pessary**. A stiff ring inserted into the vagina to help prevent urine leakage, useful in cases of a cystocele (prolapsed bladder) or rectocele.

Surgery
Your health-care professional may consider surgery to address the underlying cause of your urinary retention if other less invasive treatments are ineffective. Some surgical treatments may include:

- removing part of the prostate
- repairing urethral strictures or bladder neck scar tissue
- repairing pelvic organ prolapse
- removing a tumor, abnormal uterus, or damaged portion of a herniated disc
- repairing an abnormal bladder
- performing a urinary diversion procedure to reroute normal urine flow out of your body

CAN I PREVENT URINARY RETENTION?
While you cannot always prevent urinary retention, you can take steps to reduce your risk.

Change Your Bathroom Habits
Use the bathroom whenever you feel the urge to go. Regularly holding urine can weaken your bladder muscles and increase your risk of developing urinary tract infections (UTIs), which can lead to urinary retention.

Stay in Tune with Your Body
Monitor how often you feel the urge to urinate. If it becomes easier to delay urination and you stretch the time between bathroom visits, you may be gradually stretching your bladder. Also, note any difficulty in initiating urination or the sensation that you are unable to fully empty your bladder; these may be early signs of urinary retention.

Take Medicine as Prescribed
Men with prostate problems, such as benign prostatic hyperplasia, should adhere to the medications prescribed by their health-care professional and avoid medications that may contribute to urinary retention, such as decongestants and nonsteroidal anti-inflammatory drugs.

Do Pelvic Floor Muscle Exercises

Pelvic floor exercises, also called "Kegel exercises," can strengthen the pelvic floor muscles and improve bladder and bowel function. Both men and women can benefit from these exercises.

Make Dietary and Lifestyle Modifications

To prevent urinary retention caused by constipation, adopt dietary and lifestyle changes. Ensure an adequate intake of fiber, drink plenty of water and other liquids, and engage in regular physical activity.[1]

[1] "Urinary Retention," National Institute of Diabetes and Digestive and Kidney Diseases (NIDDK), December 2019. Available online. URL: www.niddk.nih.gov/health-information/urologic-diseases/urinary-retention/all-content. Accessed October 18, 2024.

Chapter 23 | Interstitial Cystitis

WHAT IS INTERSTITIAL CYSTITIS?

Interstitial cystitis (IC), also known as "bladder pain syndrome," is a chronic condition that causes painful urinary symptoms. Symptoms of IC may vary from person to person. Some individuals may experience mild discomfort, pressure, or tenderness in the pelvic area, while others may suffer from intense bladder pain or struggle with urinary urgency—the sudden need to urinate—and frequency—the need to urinate more often.

Health-care professionals diagnose IC by ruling out other conditions with similar symptoms.

CAUSES OF INTERSTITIAL CYSTITIS

The exact cause of IC remains unknown. Some researchers believe that IC may result from conditions that cause inflammation in various organs and parts of the body.

Severe IC symptoms can significantly affect quality of life. Individuals may feel unable to exercise or leave their homes due to frequent bathroom trips, and relationships may suffer because of painful sexual experiences.

Collaborating with health-care professionals, including a urologist or urogynecologist and a pain specialist, may help improve symptoms.

HOW COMMON IS INTERSTITIAL CYSTITIS?

Interstitial cystitis is relatively common, potentially affecting between 3 and 8 million women and between 1 and 4 million men in the United States.

WHO IS MORE LIKELY TO DEVELOP INTERSTITIAL CYSTITIS?

Interstitial cystitis can occur at any age, including childhood, but it is most prevalent in adult women and men. Approximately twice as many women are affected as men. However, recent research indicates that more men may struggle with IC than previously thought.

Some studies suggest that women are more likely to develop IC if they have a history of sexual abuse or physical trauma.

ASSOCIATED HEALTH PROBLEMS

Many women with IC are more likely to have other conditions, such as irritable bowel syndrome, fibromyalgia, and chronic fatigue syndrome. Allergies and some autoimmune diseases are also associated with IC.

Vulvodynia, which is chronic pain in the vulva often causing a burning or stinging sensation or rawness, is commonly linked to IC. Vulvodynia shares overlapping symptoms with IC.

COMPLICATIONS OF INTERSTITIAL CYSTITIS

The symptoms of IC—such as urgency, frequency, and pain—may lead individuals to reduce their physical and social activities, negatively affecting their quality of life.

Women with pelvic pain or vulvodynia often experience pain during sexual intercourse, which can damage relationships and self-image. Men may also experience pelvic pain that leads to uncomfortable or painful sexual encounters. In some cases, sexual activity can exacerbate bladder pain attacks, known as "symptom flares."

Sexual complications may cause individuals to avoid further intimacy, potentially leading to feelings of depression and guilt. Like many people dealing with chronic pain, those with IC are more likely to struggle with sleep loss due to the frequent need to urinate, as well as anxiety and depression.

Medical tests, such as pelvic exams and Pap tests, can often be painful for women with IC symptoms, particularly for those experiencing pelvic floor muscle spasms. It is important not to avoid these tests. Discuss with your health-care professional how to make pelvic exams and Pap tests more comfortable, as well as how often they should be performed.[1]

[1] "Definition and Facts of Interstitial Cystitis," National Institute of Diabetes and Digestive and Kidney Diseases (NIDDK), July 2017. Available online. URL: www.niddk.nih.gov/health-information/urologic-diseases/interstitial-cystitis-painful-bladder-syndrome/definition-facts. Accessed October 18, 2024.

Chapter 24 | Cystocele

WHAT IS A CYSTOCELE?

A cystocele is a condition in which the supportive tissues around the bladder and vaginal wall weaken and stretch, allowing the bladder and vaginal wall to fall into the vaginal canal.

Usually, the muscles and connective tissues that support the vaginal wall hold the bladder in place. With a cystocele, the muscles and tissues supporting the vagina weaken and stretch, allowing the bladder to move out of place.

A cystocele is the most common type of pelvic organ prolapse. Pelvic organ prolapse occurs when the vaginal walls, uterus, or both lose their normal support and prolapse, or bulge, into the vaginal canal or through the vaginal opening. Other nearby pelvic organs, such as the bladder or bowel, may also drop from their normal position in the body.

Health-care professionals typically rank a cystocele using a grading or staging system. Grade 1 is the mildest form of the condition, while grades 3 and 4 are the most serious. In more advanced cases of cystocele, the bladder and vaginal wall may drop far enough to reach or bulge into the vaginal canal and potentially protrude through the opening of the vagina.

WHO IS MORE LIKELY TO HAVE A CYSTOCELE?

A cystocele can affect women of any age, but the likelihood of developing one increases with age, as muscles and tissues often become weaker over time. Other factors that increase the risk of having a cystocele include:

- giving birth vaginally
- having a history of pelvic surgery, such as hysterectomy or pelvic organ prolapse repair surgery

- being overweight or having obesity
- having a family history of pelvic organ prolapse

WHAT ARE THE SYMPTOMS OF A CYSTOCELE?

Many women with cystoceles experience no symptoms. The more advanced a cystocele is, the more likely it is that symptoms will occur. Symptoms may include:

- a vaginal bulge or the sensation that something is falling out of the vagina
- pressure in the vagina or pelvis

These symptoms may worsen when straining, lifting heavy items, coughing, or standing for long periods, and they may improve when lying down.

Other symptoms may include:

- urine leakage, called "urinary incontinence"
- difficulty starting the flow of urine, called "hesitancy"
- a slow urine stream
- feeling the need to urinate after finishing urination
- frequent or urgent urination

WHAT CAUSES A CYSTOCELE?

A cystocele results from weakened or damaged muscles and connective tissues that support the bladder and vaginal walls. Multiple factors may contribute to the stretching or weakening of these muscles and tissues, including:

- pregnancy and childbirth, particularly vaginal childbirth
- conditions that repeatedly strain or increase pressure in the pelvic area, such as severe constipation, obesity, heavy lifting, or chronic cough
- prior pelvic reconstructive surgeries, such as hysterectomy or pelvic organ prolapse repair surgery
- inherited genetic factors
- certain connective tissue disorders, such as Ehlers-Danlos syndrome

HOW DO HEALTH-CARE PROFESSIONALS DIAGNOSE A CYSTOCELE?

To diagnose a cystocele, health-care professionals will ask about your symptoms and medical history and perform a physical exam, including a pelvic exam, to check your lower abdomen. You may be asked to stand during part of the exam, which may feel awkward but allows your health-care professional to determine the severity of the cystocele. Your health-care professional may also order medical tests to determine how advanced the cystocele is or to help find or rule out other problems in your urinary tract or pelvis.

HOW DO HEALTH-CARE PROFESSIONALS TREAT A CYSTOCELE?

If you do not have symptoms, your cystocele usually does not require treatment.

If you have a cystocele with symptoms, your health-care professional may recommend nonsurgical treatment or surgery, depending on the severity of the cystocele, your age, other health problems, sexual activity, desire for future children, and personal preferences.

CAN I PREVENT A CYSTOCELE?

While a cystocele usually cannot be prevented, you can take steps to relieve symptoms and help prevent the condition from worsening.

- **Do pelvic floor muscle exercises**. Strong pelvic floor muscles help hold the pelvic organs in place. Kegel exercises can strengthen the pelvic floor muscles.
- **Maintain a healthy weight**. Being overweight puts pressure on your pelvis. Make changes to your diet and lifestyle, such as eating more fruits and vegetables and getting regular physical activity.
- **Avoid heavy lifting and lift correctly**. When lifting heavy objects, use your legs instead of your waist or back.

- **Prevent and treat constipation**. Get enough fiber in your diet, drink plenty of water and other liquids, and engage in regular physical activity.
- **Control chronic cough**. Seek treatment for a chronic cough or bronchitis, and avoid smoking.[1]

[1] "Cystocele," National Institute of Diabetes and Digestive and Kidney Diseases (NIDDK), August 2020. Available online. URL: www.niddk.nih.gov/health-information/urologic-diseases/cystocele. Accessed October 18, 2024.

Chapter 25 | Bladder Cancer

WHAT IS BLADDER CANCER?

Bladder cancer occurs when cells in the bladder start to grow uncontrollably. The bladder is a hollow, balloon-shaped organ located in the lower part of the abdomen that stores urine.

The bladder has a muscular wall that allows it to enlarge to store urine produced by the kidneys and to contract to expel urine from the body. The kidneys, two organs situated above the waist on either side of the backbone, work together with the bladder to eliminate toxins and wastes from the body through urine:

- Tiny tubules in the kidneys filter and clean the blood.
- These tubules remove waste products and produce urine.
- The urine passes from each kidney through a long tube called a "ureter" into the bladder.
- The bladder holds the urine until it is expelled through a tube called the "urethra," which carries urine out of the body.

TYPES OF BLADDER CANCER

Urothelial carcinoma (also called "transitional cell carcinoma") is cancer that begins in the urothelial cells, which line the urethra, bladder, ureters, renal pelvis, and some other organs. Almost all bladder cancers are urothelial carcinomas.

Urothelial cells are also referred to as "transitional cells" because they can change shape. These cells are able to stretch when the bladder is full and shrink when it is emptied.

Other types of bladder cancer are rare:

- **Squamous cell carcinoma begins in squamous cells (thin, flat cells lining the inside of the bladder).** This type of cancer may develop after long-term irritation or infection from a tropical parasite called "schistosomiasis," which is common in Africa and the Middle East but rare in the United States. Chronic irritation can gradually transform transitional cells that line the bladder into squamous cells.
- **Adenocarcinoma begins in glandular cells found in the bladder's lining.** These glandular cells produce mucus and other substances.
- **Small cell carcinoma of the bladder originates in neuroendocrine cells.** These are nerve-like cells that release hormones into the blood in response to signals from the nervous system.

Bladder cancer can also be categorized in other ways:

- Nonmuscle-invasive bladder cancer is cancer that has not penetrated the muscle wall of the bladder. Most bladder cancers fall into this category.
- Muscle-invasive bladder cancer has spread through the lining of the bladder and into the muscle wall or beyond.

BLADDER CANCER SYMPTOMS

The symptoms of bladder cancer can vary from person to person. The most common symptom is blood in the urine, called "hematuria," which may appear slightly rusty to bright red in color. Blood may be visible at one time and not at another, and sometimes very small amounts of blood can only be detected through testing.

Other common symptoms of bladder cancer include:

- frequent urination
- pain or burning during urination
- feeling an urgent need to urinate even if the bladder is not full
- urinating often during the night

When the cancer has grown large or spread beyond the bladder to other parts of the body, additional symptoms may include:

- inability to urinate
- lower back pain on one side of the body
- abdominal pain
- bone pain or tenderness
- unintended weight loss and loss of appetite
- swelling in the feet
- fatigue

BLADDER CANCER CAUSES AND RISK FACTORS

Bladder cancer results from changes in how bladder cells function, particularly how they grow and divide. While there are many risk factors for bladder cancer, not all directly cause the disease; instead, they increase the likelihood of DNA damage in cells that may lead to cancer.

A risk factor is anything that increases the likelihood of developing a disease. Some risk factors for bladder cancer, such as tobacco use, are modifiable, while others, such as age and family history, are not. Understanding these risk factors is important for making informed decisions that could potentially lower the risk of developing bladder cancer.

In the United States, bladder cancer occurs more frequently in men than in women and more often in white individuals than in Black individuals. It can be diagnosed at any age, but the risk increases with age.

- Tobacco use, particularly smoking cigarettes, is a major risk factor for bladder cancer. Tobacco contains harmful chemicals called "carcinogens," which get absorbed into the bloodstream, filtered by the kidneys, and collected in the urine, exposing the bladder to high levels of these chemicals that can damage DNA in the bladder cells.

Other risk factors for bladder cancer include:

- family history of bladder cancer
- certain genetic changes linked to bladder cancer

- exposure to paints, dyes, metals, or petroleum products in the workplace
- prior treatment with radiation therapy to the pelvis or with certain anticancer drugs, such as cyclophosphamide or ifosfamide
- consumption of the Chinese herb *Aristolochia fangchi*
- drinking water from wells with high arsenic levels
- consumption of water treated with chlorine
- bladder infection caused by the parasite *Schistosoma haematobium*, common in Africa and the Middle East but rare in the United States
- prolonged use of urinary catheters

BLADDER CANCER DIAGNOSIS

If you exhibit symptoms or lab test results suggestive of bladder cancer, your doctor will investigate whether they are due to cancer or another condition. Your doctor may:

- inquire about your personal and family medical history to learn more about your symptoms and potential risk factors for bladder cancer
- request a urine sample for lab analysis to check for blood, abnormal cells, or infection
- conduct a physical exam, which for women may include a pelvic exam, to look for signs of cancer

Depending on your symptoms, medical history, and urine lab test results, your doctor may recommend additional tests to determine whether you have bladder cancer and, if so, its stage.

GETTING A SECOND OPINION

Some individuals may wish to obtain a second opinion to confirm their bladder cancer diagnosis and treatment plan. If you choose to seek a second opinion, you will need to provide the second doctor with important medical test results and reports from the first doctor. The second doctor will review the pathology report, slides, and scans before making a recommendation. The second opinion may align with the first doctor's conclusion, suggest modifications or alternative approaches, or provide additional insights regarding your cancer.

BLADDER CANCER TREATMENT

Various treatment options are available for bladder cancer. You and your cancer care team will collaborate to develop a treatment plan, which may encompass multiple types of treatments. Key factors considered include the stage and grade of the cancer, your overall health, and your preferences. Your treatment plan will outline details about your cancer, treatment goals, options available, possible side effects, and the expected duration of treatment.

COPING WITH BLADDER CANCER

Upon receiving a bladder cancer diagnosis, you may feel overwhelmed by the impending changes in your life. It is beneficial to familiarize yourself with the physical and emotional changes you may encounter and to identify resources available to assist you. Discussing your concerns with your health-care team can provide a greater sense of control. Additionally, family and friends can be vital sources of support.

When a child is diagnosed with cancer, every family member requires support. Taking care of yourself during this challenging time is essential. Seek assistance from your child's treatment team and the people in your family and community.[1]

[1] "What Is Bladder Cancer?" National Cancer Institute (NCI), February 16, 2023. Available online. URL: www.cancer.gov/types/bladder. Accessed October 25, 2024.

Chapter 26 | Prostate Cancer

WHAT IS THE PROSTATE?

The prostate is a part of the male reproductive system, which includes the penis, prostate, seminal vesicles, and testicles. The prostate is located just below the bladder and in front of the rectum (see Figure 26.1). It is about the size of a walnut and surrounds the urethra (the tube that empties urine from the bladder). It produces fluid that makes up a part of semen.

As a man ages, the prostate tends to increase in size. This can cause the urethra to narrow and decrease urine flow. This is called "benign prostatic hyperplasia," and it is not the same as prostate cancer. Men may also have other prostate changes that are not cancer.

SYMPTOMS OF PROSTATE CANCER

Different people have different symptoms for prostate cancer. Most men do not have symptoms at all.

If you have any of the following symptoms, be sure to see your doctor right away:

- difficulty starting urination
- weak or interrupted flow of urine
- urinating often, especially at night
- trouble emptying the bladder completely
- pain or burning during urination
- blood in the urine or semen
- pain in the back, hips, or pelvis that does not go away
- painful ejaculation

Keep in mind that these symptoms may be caused by conditions other than prostate cancer.

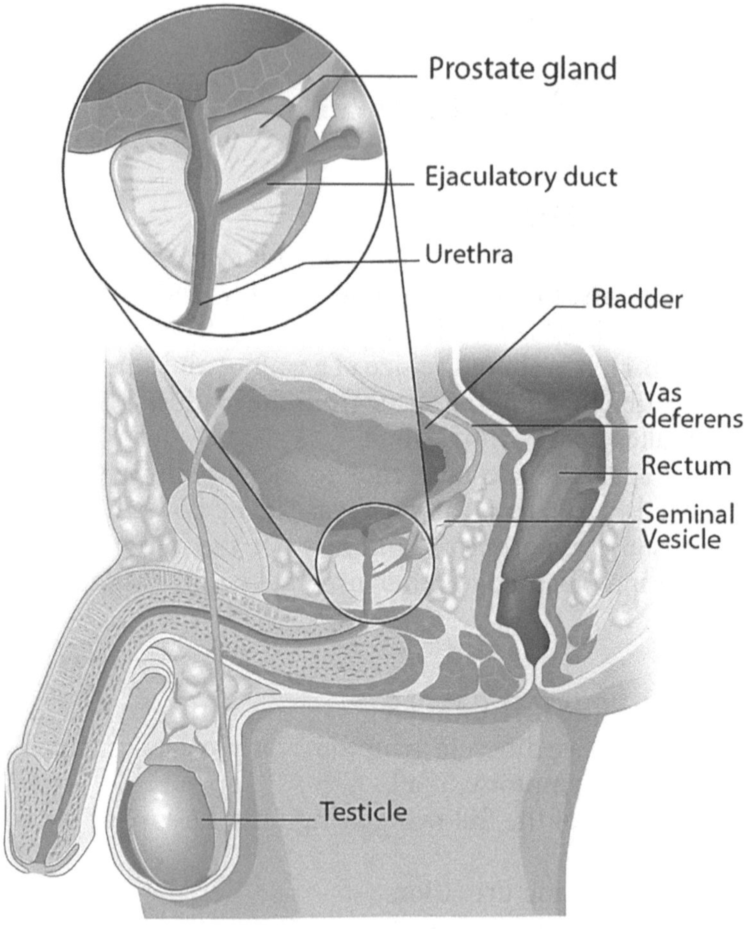

Figure 26.1. Anatomical Location of the Prostate Gland

Centers for Disease Control and Prevention (CDC)

PROSTATE CANCER RISK FACTORS

All men are at risk for prostate cancer. The most common risk factor is age.

Conditions That Can Increase Risk

All men are at risk for prostate cancer. Out of every 100 American men, about 13 will get prostate cancer during their lifetime, and about 2–3 men will die from prostate cancer.

The most common risk factor is age. The older a man is, the greater the chance of getting prostate cancer.

Some men are at increased risk for prostate cancer. You are at increased risk of getting or dying from prostate cancer if you are African American or have a family history of prostate cancer.

African-American men:

- are more likely to get prostate cancer than other men
- are more than twice as likely to die from prostate cancer than other men
- get prostate cancer at a younger age and tend to have more advanced disease when it is found

Family History (Genetic Risk Factors)

For some men, genetic factors may put them at higher risk of prostate cancer. You may have an increased risk of getting a type of prostate cancer caused by genetic changes that are inherited if:

- you have a first-degree relative (father, son, or brother) who had prostate cancer, including relatives in three generations on your mother's or father's side of the family
- you were diagnosed with prostate cancer when you were 55 years old or younger
- you were diagnosed with prostate cancer, and other members of your family have been diagnosed with breast, ovarian, or pancreatic cancer

Talk to your doctor about your family's health history.

DIAGNOSING PROSTATE CANCER

A biopsy is the main tool for diagnosing prostate cancer. If prostate cancer is diagnosed, other tests are done to find out if cancer cells have spread within the prostate or to other parts of the body.

Biopsy

A biopsy is a procedure that can be used to diagnose prostate cancer. A biopsy is when a small piece of tissue is removed from the prostate and looked at under a microscope to see if there are cancer cells.

A Gleason grade group is determined when the biopsy tissue is looked at under the microscope. If there is cancer, the grade indicates how likely it is to spread. The grade group ranges from 1 to 5. The lower the grade group, the less likely it is that the cancer will spread.

A biopsy is the main tool for diagnosing prostate cancer, but a doctor can use other tools to help make sure the biopsy is made in the right place. For example, doctors may use transrectal ultrasound or magnetic resonance imaging (MRI) to help guide the biopsy. With transrectal ultrasound, a probe the size of a finger is inserted into the rectum and high-energy sound waves (ultrasound) are bounced off the prostate to create a picture of the prostate called a "sonogram." MRI uses magnets and radio waves to produce images on a computer. MRI does not use any radiation.

Staging

If prostate cancer is diagnosed, other tests are done to find out if cancer cells have spread within the prostate or to other parts of the body. This process is called "staging." Whether the cancer is only in the prostate or has spread outside the prostate determines your stage of prostate cancer. The stage of prostate cancer tells doctors what kind of treatment you need.

TREATMENT OF PROSTATE CANCER

Different types of treatment are available for prostate cancer. You and your doctor will decide which treatment is right for you.

Expectant Management

If your doctor thinks your prostate cancer is unlikely to grow quickly, he or she may recommend that you do not treat the cancer right away. Instead, you can choose to wait and see if you get symptoms in one of two ways:

- **Active surveillance**. Closely monitoring prostate cancer by performing prostate-specific antigen (PSA)

tests and prostate biopsies regularly and treating the cancer only if it grows or causes symptoms.
- **Watchful waiting.** No tests are done. Your doctor treats any symptoms when they develop. This is usually recommended for men who are not expected to live for more than 10 years.

Surgery
A prostatectomy is an operation where doctors remove the prostate. Radical prostatectomy removes the prostate as well as the seminal vesicles (glands that produce the fluids that will turn into semen).

Radiation Therapy
Using high-energy rays (similar to x-rays) to kill the cancer. There are two types of radiation therapy:
- **External radiation therapy.** A machine outside the body directs radiation at the cancer cells.
- **Internal radiation therapy (brachytherapy).** Radioactive seeds or pellets are surgically placed into or near the cancer to destroy the cancer cells.

Other Therapies
Other therapies may be used, depending on whether the prostate cancer has spread:
- **Cryotherapy.** Placing a special probe inside or near the prostate cancer to freeze and kill the cancer cells. This is a less common treatment.
- **Chemotherapy.** Using special drugs to shrink or kill the cancer after it has spread to other parts of the body. The drugs can be pills you take or medicines given through your veins, or, sometimes, both.
- **Biological therapy.** Works with your body's immune system to help it fight cancer or to control side effects from other cancer treatments. Side effects are how your body reacts to drugs or other treatments.
- **High-intensity focused ultrasound.** It is a less common treatment that directs high-energy sound waves (ultrasound) at the cancer to kill cancer cells.

- **Hormone therapy**. Blocks cancer cells from getting the hormones they need to grow. This is also called "androgen deprivation therapy" (ADT).
- **Targeted therapy**. Using drugs that attack cancer cells while minimizing damage to healthy cells. Targeted therapy is used to treat prostate cancer that has spread to other parts of the body and is no longer responding to hormone therapy.[1]

[1] "Prostate Cancer Basics," Centers for Disease Control and Prevention (CDC), August 27, 2024. Available online. URL: www.cdc.gov/prostate-cancer/about/index.html. Accessed October 18, 2024.

Part 5 | Diagnostic Tests for Kidney Disease

Chapter 27 | Essential Tests for Chronic Kidney Disease Detection

Chronic kidney disease (CKD) happens when your kidneys become damaged over time and cannot filter your blood as well. Diabetes is a leading cause of CKD, and there are often no symptoms until your kidneys are badly damaged.

If you find and treat kidney disease early, you may be able to manage CKD and prevent other health complications. However, the only way to know how well your kidneys are working is to get tested.

URINE TESTS

One of the earliest signs of kidney disease is when protein leaks into your urine (proteinuria). Urine testing can check for this. There are two types of urine tests that can check your protein levels.

Dipstick Urine Test

A dipstick is a chemically treated paper placed in your urine sample. It changes color if your levels are above normal. This test is often done as part of overall urine testing, but it can also be done as a quick test to look for albumin (a protein produced by your liver) in your urine.

A dipstick urine test does not provide an exact measurement of albumin but does let your doctor know if your levels are normal. If you have abnormal albumin levels, your doctor may want to run further tests.

Urine Albumin-to-Creatinine Ratio Test

The urine albumin-to-creatinine ratio (UACR) test measures the amount of albumin and compares it to the amount of creatinine (a normal waste product from your muscles) in your urine. A UACR test lets the doctor know how much albumin passes into your urine over a 24-hour period. A urine albumin test result of 30 or above may mean kidney disease.

It is important to know that:

- The test may be repeated once or twice to confirm the results.
- If you have kidney disease, your albumin level in your urine helps your doctor determine the best treatment option.
- If your urine albumin level stays the same or goes down, it means your treatment is working.

SERUM CREATININE

Because your kidneys remove waste, toxins, and extra fluid from the blood, blood tests can check your kidney function. They will show how well and how quickly your kidneys are doing their job to remove waste.

A serum creatinine blood test measures the amount of creatinine in your blood. If your kidneys are not working well, your creatinine level goes up. Normal levels for you will depend on your sex, age, and muscle mass.

A creatinine level of more than 1.2 for women and 1.4 for men may usually indicate that the kidneys are not working well.

GLOMERULAR FILTRATION RATE

The glomerular filtration rate (GFR) is a blood test that measures how well your kidneys remove waste, toxins, and extra fluid from your blood. Your serum creatinine level, age, and sex are used to calculate your GFR number. Like other kidney tests, a normal GFR number for you will depend on your age and sex.

If your GFR is low, your kidneys are likely not working as they should. As kidney disease progresses, your GFR goes down. The results of your test can mean the following:

- **If your GFR is 60 or more, together with a normal urine albumin test, you are in the normal range.** However, you will still want to talk to your doctor about when you should be checked again.

- **If your GFR is less than 60, you may have kidney disease.** Talk to your doctor about the best treatment options for you.
- **If your GFR is less than 15, it may mean your kidneys are failing.** If your results show kidney failure, you will likely need dialysis or a kidney transplant. If your GFR level is less than 20 over 6–12 months, your doctor may consider a kidney transplant.

BLOOD UREA NITROGEN

A blood urea nitrogen (BUN) is a blood test that measures the amount of urea nitrogen in your blood. Urea nitrogen is a waste product your body makes from the breakdown of protein in the foods you eat. Healthy kidneys filter urea nitrogen out of your blood, which leaves your body through your urine. This process helps keep your BUN level within a normal range.

A normal BUN level depends on your age and other health conditions but usually ranges from 7 to 20. If your BUN level is higher than normal, this may be a sign that your kidneys are not working well. As kidney disease progresses, your BUN level goes up.

OTHER TESTS

Your doctor may also perform other tests to check your kidneys. These could include monitoring your blood pressure, running imaging tests, or performing a kidney biopsy. Kidney testing helps you and your doctor determine the best treatment plan for you.[1]

[1] "Testing for Chronic Kidney Disease," Centers for Disease Control and Prevention (CDC), May 15, 2024. Available online. URL: www.cdc.gov/kidney-disease/testing/index.html. Accessed October 19, 2024.

Chapter 28 | **Blood Tests for Kidney Function**

Chapter Contents

WHAT IS A CREATININE TEST?

The creatinine test measures creatinine levels in a blood and/or urine sample. Creatinine is a normal waste product in the body made when muscles are used and some muscle tissue breaks down.

Normally, your kidneys filter creatinine from your blood and remove it from your body in your urine. If there is a problem with your kidneys, creatinine can build up in your blood, and less may be released in urine. If blood and/or urine creatinine levels are not normal, it may be a sign of kidney disease.

Creatinine in blood may be measured by itself or as part of a group of tests called a "comprehensive metabolic panel" (CMP) or a "basic metabolic panel" (BMP). Your health-care provider may order these tests as part of a routine checkup.

WHAT IS IT USED FOR?

A creatinine test is used to help with the following:

- Check the health of your kidneys.
- Diagnose kidney disease.
- Monitor known kidney problems and see how well treatment is working.
- Check for side effects from medicines that may affect your kidneys.

Creatinine testing alone is not the best way to check how well your kidneys are working. This is because people produce different amounts of creatinine depending on how much muscle they have, the foods they eat, their age, and how active they are. Therefore, the results from creatinine testing are often used in calculations or compared with other substances to help provide more information:

- **Estimated glomerular filtration rate (eGFR).** Creatinine levels in blood are often used to calculate how fast your kidneys filter waste out of your blood.

This calculation includes information about your age, weight, height, and sex. An eGFR is a more accurate way to measure kidney health than creatinine levels in blood or urine alone. An eGFR can also help show how serious kidney disease may be.

- **Creatinine clearance calculation**. Creatinine levels in blood and urine may be compared with each other. This helps estimate how fast your kidneys filter waste. However, an eGFR is more accurate. A creatinine clearance may still be useful to help identify the cause of high or low levels of blood creatinine in people with very high muscle mass or a loss of muscle mass from age, illness, or the loss of an arm and/or leg.
- **Urine albumin to creatinine ratio (UACR)**. Creatinine levels in urine may be used to calculate a urine albumin to creatinine ratio (UACR), which is sometimes called a "microalbumin creatinine ratio." Albumin is the main protein found in the blood. Normally, your kidneys filter out just a trace of albumin, or none at all. If larger amounts of albumin pass into your urine, it may be a sign of kidney damage. A UACR compares the amounts of creatinine and albumin in your urine to get a more accurate measurement of how much albumin is in your urine.
- **Blood urea nitrogen (BUN)**. Creatinine blood levels measured as part of a CMP or a BMP may be compared with the level of BUN measured in the same test. This can help determine the cause of a kidney problem.

WHY DO I NEED IT?

Your provider may order a creatinine test:

- to check your kidney health as part of a routine checkup
- if you have symptoms of kidney disease, which may include:
  - swelling in the hands and feet or puffy eyelids
  - dry skin, itching, or numbness
  - fatigue

- increased or decreased need to urinate
- urine that is bloody or foamy
- loss of appetite and weight loss
- muscle cramps
- nausea and vomiting
- shortness of breath
- sleep problems
- trouble thinking clearly

If you have a high risk of developing kidney disease, even if you do not have symptoms now. Chronic (long-term) kidney disease (CKD) often does not have symptoms in the early stages. Your risk for kidney disease is increased if you:

- have diabetes
- have high blood pressure (HBP)
- have a family health history of kidney disease, diabetes, or HBP
- have heart disease
- are over 50 years old
- smoke
- have obesity

If you have kidney problems or possible kidney problems because you:

- had an abnormal result on a kidney test in the past
- have been diagnosed with kidney disease
- have taken certain medicines that could affect your kidneys
- have had a kidney transplant

WHAT HAPPENS DURING THE TEST?

For a Creatinine Blood Test

A health-care professional will take a blood sample from a vein in your arm using a small needle. After the needle is inserted, a small amount of blood will be collected into a test tube or vial. You may feel a little sting when the needle goes in or out. This usually takes less than five minutes.

For a Creatinine Urine Test

You may need to provide all the urine you pass over 24 hours, as creatinine levels vary throughout the day. However, your provider may use a urine sample for a shorter period of time.

For a 24-hour urine sample, you will be given a special container to collect your urine over a full day and instructions on how to collect and store your sample. Your provider will tell you what time to start. The test generally includes the following steps:

1. To begin, urinate in the toilet as usual. Do not collect this urine. Write down the time you urinated.
2. For the next 24 hours, collect all your urine in the container.
3. During the collection period, store the urine container in a refrigerator or in a cooler with ice.
4. Try to urinate 24 hours after starting the test. This is the last urine collection for the test.
5. Return the container with your urine to your provider's office or the laboratory as instructed.

WILL I NEED TO DO ANYTHING TO PREPARE FOR THE TEST?

Your provider will let you know how to prepare for your test. You may be told to avoid eating meat for 24 hours before your test, as meat can temporarily increase creatinine levels.

If creatinine is being measured as part of a CMP or a BMP test, you may need to fast (not eat or drink) for up to 12 hours before your test.

Certain medicines and supplements can affect your test results, so be sure to tell your provider everything you are taking. However, do not stop taking any medicine unless your provider tells you to stop.

WHAT DO THE RESULTS MEAN?

Normal

Creatinine levels that are considered normal for you will depend on how much muscle you have, what you eat, your age, and how active you are. If you are healthy, your levels are usually fairly stable over time.

However, a normal creatinine test result does not always mean that your kidneys are healthy. Sometimes, blood creatinine levels remain in a normal range during the early stages of kidney disease.

They rise as the condition of your kidneys becomes more serious. If your provider suspects you have a kidney condition, you will likely have other kidney tests even if your creatinine results seem normal.

Abnormal

If your results are abnormal, a single high creatinine test cannot diagnose a specific condition. You will likely need to be retested and/or have other tests as well.

High

In general, if your blood creatinine level is high for you, it may be a sign of:

- kidney disease or injury, including infection, poor blood flow to the kidneys, a blockage in the urinary system, or kidney failure
- a condition that affects your kidneys, such as heart failure or diabetes

High blood creatinine levels do not always mean you have a kidney problem. They may be caused by dehydration, muscle disorders and injuries, muscular dystrophy, intense exercise, or a diet high in meat. Certain health problems in pregnancy can also cause increases in creatinine.

Low

In general, if your blood creatinine level is low for you, it may be a sign of:

- malnutrition or a condition that causes your muscles to get smaller, such as a long illness, a nerve disorder, or muscle loss from aging

Serious liver disease can also lead to low levels. Low levels of blood creatinine are not common.

If you have questions about any of your results, talk with your provider.[1]

---

[1] MedlinePlus, "Creatinine Test," National Institutes of Health (NIH), December 5, 2023. Available online. URL: https://medlineplus.gov/lab-tests/creatinine-test. Accessed October 19, 2024.

Section 28.2 | **Blood Urea Nitrogen Test**

WHAT IS A BLOOD UREA NITROGEN TEST?

A blood urea nitrogen (BUN) test can provide important information about kidney function. The main job of the kidneys is to remove waste and extra fluid from the body. If kidney disease is present, waste material can build up in the blood, potentially leading to serious health problems, including high blood pressure (HBP), anemia, and heart disease.

The BUN test measures the amount of urea nitrogen in the blood. Urea nitrogen is a waste product that the kidneys remove from the blood. Higher-than-normal BUN levels may indicate that the kidneys are not functioning well.

People with early kidney disease may not exhibit any symptoms. A BUN test can help uncover kidney problems at an early stage when treatment can be more effective.

WHAT IS IT USED FOR?

A BUN test is often part of a series of tests called a "comprehensive metabolic panel." It can help diagnose or monitor kidney disease or disorders.

WHY DO I NEED IT?

Your health-care provider may order a BUN test as part of a routine checkup or if you have or are at risk for a kidney problem. Early kidney disease typically does not present any signs or symptoms. You may be more likely to develop kidney disease if you have:

- a family history of kidney problems
- diabetes
- high blood pressure
- heart disease

Your provider may check your BUN levels if you are experiencing symptoms of later-stage kidney disease, such as:

- needing to urinate more or less often than usual
- itching

- fatigue
- swelling in your legs, feet, or ankles
- muscle cramps
- trouble sleeping

WHAT HAPPENS DURING THE TEST?

A health-care professional will take a blood sample from a vein in your arm using a small needle. After the needle is inserted, a small amount of blood will be collected into a test tube or vial. You may feel a little sting when the needle goes in or out. This procedure usually takes less than five minutes.

WILL I NEED TO DO ANYTHING TO PREPARE FOR THE TEST?

Usually, there is no special preparation necessary for a BUN test. However, if your provider has ordered other tests on your blood sample, you may need to fast (not eat or drink) for several hours before the test.

WHAT DO THE RESULTS MEAN?

Normal

Normal BUN levels can vary, but generally, a high level of blood urea nitrogen is a sign that the kidneys are not functioning well. However, abnormal results do not always indicate that a medical condition requires treatment.

High

Higher-than-normal BUN levels can also be caused by dehydration (too little fluid in the body), burns, certain medications, a high-protein diet, or other factors, including age. BUN levels typically increase with age. To learn what your results mean, discuss them with your health-care provider.[1]

[1] MedlinePlus, "BUN (Blood Urea Nitrogen)," National Institutes of Health (NIH), April 5, 2022. Available online. URL: https://medlineplus.gov/lab-tests/bun-blood-urea-nitrogen. Accessed October 19, 2024.

Section 28.3 | Renal Panel Tests

A test in which blood or urine samples are checked for the amounts of certain substances released by the kidneys. A higher- or lower-than-normal amount of a substance can be a sign that the kidneys are not working the way they should. Also called "kidney function test." The kidney function tests are vital for assessing kidney health and diagnosing related conditions by measuring key substances in the blood. These tests help detect electrolyte imbalances, monitor kidney disease, and ensure proper acid-base balance for overall metabolic health.[1]

ALBUMIN BLOOD TEST

What Is an Albumin Blood Test?

An albumin blood test measures the amount of albumin in the blood. Low albumin levels can be a sign of liver or kidney disease or another medical condition, while high levels may indicate dehydration.

Albumin is a protein made by the liver. It enters the bloodstream and helps keep fluid from leaking out of blood vessels into other tissues. It also carries hormones, vitamins, and enzymes throughout the body. Without enough albumin, fluid can leak out of the blood and build up in the lungs, abdomen, or other parts of the body.

- **Other names**: ALB; serum albumin test.

What Is It Used For?

An albumin blood test is used to check general health and assess the liver and kidneys' functioning. If the liver is damaged or not well nourished, it may not produce enough albumin. If the kidneys are damaged, they may allow too much albumin to leave the body in urine.

An albumin blood test is often conducted as part of a group of blood tests measuring different enzymes, proteins, and other substances made in the liver. These tests are called "liver function tests" or "liver panel". An albumin test may also be part of a comprehensive

[1] "Renal Function Test," National Cancer Institute (NCI), September 13, 2016. Available online. URL: www.cancer.gov/publications/dictionaries/cancer-terms/def/renal-function-test. Accessed October 19, 2024.

metabolic panel (CMP), a group of routine blood tests that measure several substances.[2]

ANION GAP BLOOD TEST

What Is an Anion Gap Blood Test?

An anion gap blood test checks the acid-base balance (pH balance) of the blood. It indicates if the blood is too acidic or not acidic enough. The test uses results from another blood test called an "electrolyte panel." Electrolytes are electrically charged minerals in the body, such as sodium, potassium, and bicarbonate, that help control the acid-base balance of the blood.

Some electrolytes have a positive electric charge, while others have a negative electric charge. The anion gap measures the difference—or gap—between the negatively charged and positively charged electrolytes in the blood. If the anion gap is too high, the blood is more acidic than normal. If the anion gap is too low, the blood is not acidic enough. Both high and low results may indicate a serious disorder that needs attention.

- **Other name**: Serum anion gap.

What Is It Used For?

The anion gap blood test indicates whether electrolytes are out of balance or if the blood is too acidic or not acidic enough. Excess acid in the blood is termed "acidosis," while insufficient acid is called "alkalosis." Both conditions can be serious.[3]

CARBON DIOXIDE BLOOD TEST

What Is a Carbon Dioxide Blood Test?

A carbon dioxide (CO_2) blood test measures the amount of CO_2 in the blood. CO_2 is an odorless, colorless gas that is a waste product produced when the body uses food for energy.

[2] MedlinePlus, "Albumin Blood Test," National Institutes of Health (NIH), June 7, 2022. Available online. URL: https://medlineplus.gov/lab-tests/albumin-blood-test. Accessed October 19, 2024.
[3] MedlinePlus, "Anion Gap Blood Test," National Institutes of Health (NIH), April 7, 2022. Available online. URL: https://medlineplus.gov/lab-tests/anion-gap-blood-test. Accessed October 19, 2024.

Blood carries CO_2 to the lungs, where it is exhaled. Abnormal levels of CO_2 in the blood can indicate a health problem.

- **Other names**: Carbon dioxide content; CO_2 content; carbon dioxide blood test; bicarbonate blood test; bicarbonate test; total CO_2; bicarb; HCO_3.

What Is It Used For?

Most of the CO_2 in the body is bicarbonate, a type of electrolyte that helps control fluid balance and the balance of acids and bases (pH balance). A CO_2 blood test is often part of an electrolyte panel, which may be included in routine check-ups. The test helps diagnose or monitor conditions related to electrolyte imbalances, such as high blood pressure and diseases of the kidneys, lungs, or liver.[4]

CHLORIDE BLOOD TEST

What Is a Chloride Blood Test?

A chloride blood test measures the amount of chloride in the blood. Chloride is a type of electrolyte that helps control fluid balance and the balance of acids and bases (pH balance) in the body. Chloride is often measured with other electrolytes to diagnose or monitor conditions such as kidney disease, heart failure, liver disease, and high blood pressure.

- **Other names**: CI; serum chloride.

What Is It Used For?

A chloride test is typically included in a routine blood screening to check general health and diagnose conditions related to imbalances of acids or fluids in the body.[5]

[4] MedlinePlus, "Carbon Dioxide (CO_2) in Blood," National Institutes of Health (NIH), August 3, 2022. Available online. URL: https://medlineplus.gov/lab-tests/carbon-dioxide-co2-in-blood. Accessed October 19, 2024.
[5] MedlinePlus, "Chloride Blood Test," National Institutes of Health (NIH), April 8, 2022. Available online. URL: https://medlineplus.gov/lab-tests/chloride-blood-test. Accessed October 19, 2024.

MAGNESIUM BLOOD TEST

What Is a Magnesium Blood Test?

A magnesium blood test measures the amount of magnesium in a sample of blood. Magnesium is a mineral obtained from various foods, such as nuts, seeds, beans, fortified cereals, leafy greens, and milk.

The body needs magnesium for proper muscle, nerve, and heart function. Magnesium also helps control blood pressure and blood glucose levels and is essential for building strong bones and supporting the immune system.

Magnesium is an electrolyte that helps control fluid balance and the balance of acids and bases (pH balance) in the body. Most of the body's magnesium is stored in bones, organs, and tissues, with only a small amount found in blood.

Abnormal blood magnesium levels can be caused by various conditions, so a magnesium test may be used to diagnose a variety of disorders.

- **Other names**: Mg; Mag; Magnesium-Serum.

What Is It Used For?

A magnesium blood test checks the level of magnesium in the blood. It is performed if the health-care provider suspects abnormal levels:

- **Low magnesium level.** Hypomagnesemia, more common than elevated levels.
- **High magnesium level.** Hypermagnesemia, which is uncommon and usually occurs in people with kidney failure.

A magnesium blood test may also help identify the cause of abnormal levels of other minerals, including calcium, potassium, and phosphorus, as magnesium plays a role in the absorption of these minerals.[6]

[6] MedlinePlus, "Magnesium Blood Test," National Institutes of Health (NIH), October 25, 2023. Available online. https://medlineplus.gov/lab-tests/magnesium-blood-test. Accessed October 19, 2024.

PHOSPHATE IN BLOOD TEST

What Is a Phosphate in Blood Test?

A phosphate in blood test measures the amount of phosphate in a sample of blood. Phosphate contains the mineral phosphorus, so a phosphate test is sometimes called a "phosphorus test."

Phosphate is an electrolyte that helps control fluid balance and the balance of acids and bases (pH balance) in the body. It is essential for building strong bones and teeth, making energy, and enabling proper nerve and muscle function.

The phosphorus in phosphate comes from foods such as nuts, seeds, dairy products, dried beans, meats, poultry, and eggs. The body tightly regulates phosphate levels mainly through the kidneys and intestines.

Abnormal phosphate levels may indicate issues with the systems controlling phosphate levels, and the test is often conducted alongside other tests measuring calcium, vitamin D, and parathyroid hormone (PTH).

- **Other names**: Phosphorus test; P; PO_4; phosphorus-serum; phosphate; inorganic phosphorus.

What Is It Used For?

A phosphate in blood test is often used with other tests to help diagnose or monitor:

- **Kidney disease, particularly chronic kidney disease**. High phosphate levels indicate that the kidneys are not functioning well.
- **Bone disorders**. High phosphate levels can weaken bones by pulling calcium from them.
- **Parathyroid disorders**. A phosphate test can help assess the function of parathyroid glands, which regulate phosphate and calcium levels in the blood.

A phosphate test may also monitor individuals with poorly controlled diabetes or signs of acid-base imbalance.[7]

[7] MedlinePlus, "Phosphate in Blood," National Institutes of Health (NIH), October 25, 2023. Available online. URL: https://medlineplus.gov/lab-tests/phosphate-in-blood. Accessed October 19, 2024.

SODIUM BLOOD TEST

What Is a Sodium Blood Test?

A sodium blood test measures the amount of sodium in the blood. Sodium is an electrolyte that helps control fluid balance and the balance of acids and bases (pH balance) in the body, as well as supports proper nerve and muscle function.

Most sodium intake comes from the diet. If too much sodium is consumed, the kidneys eliminate the excess sodium through urine. The body typically maintains sodium levels within a narrow range. Abnormal sodium levels may indicate kidney problems, dehydration, or other medical conditions.

Other name: Na test.

What Is It Used For?

A sodium blood test is a routine test that checks general health and helps find or monitor conditions affecting fluid balance, electrolytes, and acidity in the body. The test is often included in an electrolyte panel or as part of a basic metabolic panel (BMP) and comprehensive metabolic panel (CMP).[8]

---

[8] MedlinePlus, "Sodium Blood Test," National Institutes of Health (NIH), June 2, 2022. Available online. URL: https://medlineplus.gov/lab-tests/sodium-blood-test. Accessed October 19, 2024.

Chapter 29 | Urine Tests for Kidney Function

Chapter Contents

Section 29.1 | Calcium in Urine Test

WHAT IS A CALCIUM IN URINE TEST?

A calcium in urine test measures the amount of calcium in your urine. If your urine calcium levels are too high or too low, it may be a sign of kidney disease, kidney stones, bone disease, a parathyroid gland disorder, or other conditions.

Calcium is one of the most important minerals in your body. Most of your calcium is stored in your bones and teeth. About 1 percent of the calcium in your body is in your blood. Having the right amount of calcium in your blood is necessary for your nerves, muscles, and heart to work properly. Normally, your kidneys filter out a small amount of calcium from your blood, which leaves your body in urine.

Checking the amount of calcium in urine can help diagnose kidney problems and other conditions that can affect calcium levels in your blood. If you have symptoms of any of these conditions, your health-care provider may order a calcium blood test, too.

WHAT IS IT USED FOR?

A calcium in urine test may be used to diagnose or monitor how well your kidneys are working. It may be used if you have symptoms of kidney stones, which are more likely to form if you have too much calcium in your urine. A calcium in urine test may also help diagnose problems with the parathyroid glands in your neck. These glands help control the amount of calcium in your body.

WHY DO I NEED IT?

You may need a calcium in urine test if you have symptoms of a kidney stone. These symptoms include:

- sharp pain in your lower abdomen (belly), back, side, or groin
- blood in your urine
- frequent need to urinate
- pain while urinating

- inability to urinate or urinating only small amounts
- cloudy or bad-smelling urine
- nausea and vomiting

WHAT HAPPENS DURING THE TEST?

You will need to collect all your urine during a 24-hour period. This is called a "24-hour urine sample test." You will be given a special container to collect your urine and instructions on how to collect and store your samples. Your provider will tell you what time to start. The test generally includes the following steps:

1. To begin, urinate in the toilet as usual. Do not collect this urine. Write down the time you urinated.
2. For the next 24 hours, collect all your urine in the container.
3. During the collection period, store the urine container in a refrigerator or in a cooler with ice.
4. Try to urinate 24 hours after starting the test. This is the last urine collection for the test.
5. Return the container with your urine to your provider's office or the laboratory as instructed.

WILL I NEED TO DO ANYTHING TO PREPARE FOR THE TEST?

You may be asked to avoid certain foods and medicines for several days before the test. Do not stop taking any medicines without talking with your provider. Your provider will let you know if there are any special instructions to follow.

WHAT DO THE RESULTS MEAN?

High

Higher than normal calcium levels in urine may be a sign of:

- a kidney stone
- hyperparathyroidism (too much parathyroid hormone)
- certain types of cancer, including cancer that spreads to the bones
- Paget disease of bone

- sarcoidosis
- too much vitamin D over a long period of time, usually from supplements

Low

Lower than normal calcium levels in urine may be a sign of:

- kidney disease
- hypoparathyroidism (too little parathyroid hormone)
- hypothyroidism (too little thyroid hormone)
- too little vitamin D or magnesium
- malabsorption disorder
- malnutrition

If your calcium levels are not normal, it does not always mean you have a medical condition that needs treatment. Your diet and certain supplements and medicines, including antacids, can affect your urine calcium levels. If you have questions about your results, talk with your provider.[1]

Section 29.2 | Phosphate in Urine Test

WHAT IS A PHOSPHATE IN URINE TEST?

A phosphate in urine test measures the amount of phosphate in a urine sample that you collect over a 24-hour period. Phosphate is an electrolyte. Electrolytes are electrically charged minerals. They help control the amount of fluid and the balance of acids and bases (pH balance) in your body.

Phosphate is made of the mineral phosphorus combined with oxygen. Phosphate works with the mineral calcium to build strong bones and teeth. Most of your phosphate is stored in your bones. However, phosphate is in every cell of your body, and it affects

[1] MedlinePlus, "Calcium in Urine Test," National Institutes of Health (NIH), June 7, 2022. Available online. URL: https://medlineplus.gov/lab-tests/calcium-in-urine-test. Accessed October 25, 2024.

almost everything your cells do, including how your nerves work and how your body uses energy.

Most people get more phosphate than they need from food. Your kidneys control the amount of phosphate in your blood by removing most of the extra phosphate through your urine. Your parathyroid glands in your neck make hormones that affect how much phosphate your kidneys remove.

If you have a problem with your kidneys or your parathyroid glands, the phosphate levels in your urine may be too high or too low. This can be a sign of a serious health problem.

WHAT IS IT USED FOR?

A phosphate in urine test may be used to diagnose or monitor how well your kidneys are working. It may be used if you have symptoms of kidney stones, which are more likely to form if you have too much calcium in your urine. A phosphate in urine test may also help diagnose problems with the parathyroid glands in your neck. These glands help control the amount of calcium in your body.

WHY DO I NEED IT?

You may need a phosphate in urine test if you have symptoms of a kidney stone. These symptoms include:

- sharp pain in your lower abdomen (belly), back, side, or groin
- blood in your urine
- frequent need to urinate
- pain while urinating
- inability to urinate or urinating only small amounts
- cloudy or bad-smelling urine
- nausea and vomiting

WHAT HAPPENS DURING THE TEST?

You will need to collect all your urine during a 24-hour period. This is called a "24-hour urine sample test." You will be given a special container to collect your urine and instructions on how to collect and store your samples. Your provider will tell you what time to start. The test generally includes the following steps:

1. To begin, urinate in the toilet as usual. Do not collect this urine. Write down the time you urinated.
2. For the next 24 hours, collect all your urine in the container.
3. During the collection period, store the urine container in a refrigerator or in a cooler with ice.
4. Try to urinate 24 hours after starting the test. This is the last urine collection for the test.
5. Return the container with your urine to your provider's office or the laboratory as instructed.

WILL I NEED TO DO ANYTHING TO PREPARE FOR THE TEST?

You may be asked to avoid certain foods and medicines for several days before the test. Do not stop taking any medicines without talking with your provider. Your provider will let you know if there are any special instructions to follow.

WHAT DO THE RESULTS MEAN?

Higher than normal phosphate levels in urine may be a sign of:

- a kidney stone
- hyperparathyroidism (too much parathyroid hormone)
- certain types of cancer, including cancer that spreads to the bones
- Paget disease of bone
- sarcoidosis
- too much vitamin D over a long period of time, usually from supplements

Lower than normal phosphate levels in urine may be a sign of:

- kidney disease
- hypoparathyroidism (too little parathyroid hormone)
- hypothyroidism (too little thyroid hormone)
- too little vitamin D or magnesium

- malabsorption disorder
- malnutrition

If your phosphate levels are not normal, it does not always mean you have a medical condition that needs treatment. Your diet and certain supplements and medicines, including antacids, can affect your urine phosphate levels. If you have questions about your results, talk with your provider.[1]

[1] MedlinePlus, "Phosphate in Urine," National Institutes of Health (NIH), September 12, 2022. Available online. URL: https://medlineplus.gov/lab-tests/phosphate-in-urine. Accessed October 25, 2024.

Chapter 30 | **Urinary Tract Imaging and Kidney Biopsy**

Chapter Contents

Section 30.1 | Imaging Techniques for the Urinary Tract

The urinary tract serves as the body's drainage system for removing wastes and excess fluids. It comprises two kidneys, two ureters, a bladder, and a urethra. Imaging techniques are essential for helping health-care professionals identify the causes of medical issues related to the urinary tract. These techniques include:

- x-rays
- ultrasounds
- magnetic resonance imaging (MRI) scans
- computed tomography (CT) scans
- radionuclide scans

WHAT SYMPTOMS COULD REQUIRE IMAGING OF THE URINARY TRACT?

Imaging could be required for symptoms such as:

- difficulty initiating or maintaining urination
- difficulty in emptying the bladder, known as "urinary retention"
- accidental leakage of urine, known as "bladder control problems" or "urinary incontinence"
- urinary frequency and urgency (day or night)
- recurrent urinary tract infections (UTIs)
- a single UTI in a susceptible or high-risk person, such as an infant
- pain in the abdomen, upper or lower back, or groin
- abdominal pain or mass, such as swelling in a specific part of the abdomen
- evidence of kidney failure
- blood in the urine, known as "hematuria"
- high blood pressure

WHAT ARE SOME OTHER REASONS FOR IMAGING THE URINARY TRACT?

Your health-care professional might also order urinary tract imaging to pinpoint a problem. That is important because different urinary tract problems may share the same symptoms. For example, a urinary blockage can be caused by a kidney stone or an enlarged prostate.

Imaging can also help your health-care professional identify, evaluate, follow up, and monitor problems such as:

- kidney diseases
- tumors
- small bladder capacity
- backward flow of urine, known as "vesicoureteral reflux" (VUR)
- hydronephrosis, or urine blockage, in newborns following suspicious or abnormal imaging during pregnancy

WHAT STEPS DOES YOUR HEALTH-CARE PROFESSIONAL TAKE BEFORE ORDERING IMAGING TESTS?

Before ordering imaging tests, your health-care professional will consider your general medical history, including any major illnesses or surgeries, perform a physical exam, obtain blood test results, and may ask:

- about your specific urinary tract symptoms, when they began, how often they occur, and how severe they are
- if you take any prescription or over-the-counter medicines
- how much fluid you take in each day
- about your use of alcohol and caffeine
- whether you are allergic to any foods or medicines
- whether you could be pregnant, if you are a female patient

WHAT ARE THE IMAGING TECHNIQUES?

Your health-care professional can use several different imaging techniques, depending on factors such as your general medical history and urinary tract symptoms.

X-rays

X-rays of the urinary tract can help highlight and monitor a kidney stone or tumor that could be blocking the flow of urine and causing pain.

Conventional x-rays involve some exposure to ionizing radiation, a type of radiation strong enough to damage some cells.

Two common x-ray procedures used for urinary tract imaging include:

- intravenous pyelogram (IVP) to help locate problems in the kidneys, ureters, or bladder that may be caused by urinary retention or urinary reflux
- voiding cystourethrogram (VCUG) to view images of the bladder and urethra taken while the bladder is full and during urination

Ultrasound

Ultrasound uses a hand-held device, called a "transducer," that bounces safe, painless sound waves off organs to create an image of their structure. The health-care professional can move the transducer at different angles to examine different organs.

This procedure is painless, poses no risk of radiation, requires no anesthesia, and allows you to return to daily tasks immediately.

Health-care professionals use specific types of abdominal ultrasounds to look at different parts of the urinary tract.

- Bladder ultrasound can provide information about the bladder wall, diverticula (pouches) of the bladder, bladder stones, and large tumors in the bladder.
- Kidney ultrasound can show if the kidneys are in the right place or if they have blockages, kidney stones, or tumors.

MRI Scans

Magnetic resonance imaging (MRI) takes pictures of the body's internal organs and soft tissues without using x-rays. MRI machines use radio waves and magnets to produce detailed pictures of the body's internal organs and soft tissues. During an MRI, a special dye known as a "contrast medium" may be injected into the blood before the test, usually intravenously (IV) through a vein in the hand or forearm. The dye helps the radiologist see certain areas more clearly.

- **Magnetic resonance angiography (MRA).** An MRA is a type of MRI that provides the most detailed view of kidney arteries, which are the blood vessels that supply blood to the kidneys. An MRA can also show renal artery stenosis.

- **Magnetic resonance urography (MRU).** An MRU is a type of MRI used to evaluate patients with blood in the urine, known as "hematuria." MRU is also used when following up with patients who have a history of urinary tract cancers and to identify abnormalities in patients with recurrent urinary tract infections.

CT Scans

A CT scan combines x-rays with computer technology to create three-dimensional (3D) images. These scans can show stones in the urinary tract, as well as obstructions, infections, cysts, tumors, and traumatic injuries. Imaging for urinary stone disease can be done with low or ultra-low dose CT scans.

Radionuclide Scans

A radionuclide scan, also called a "nuclear scan" or "radioisotope scan," detects small amounts of radiation after radioactive material is injected into the blood. This scan provides information about how your kidneys function and helps health-care professionals diagnose many conditions, including cancers, injuries, and infections.

- **Renal/kidney scan.** Your health-care professional might perform a renal scan to check your kidneys and urinary system. This type of exam involves injecting a small amount of radioactive material into the blood and using a special camera and computer.

There are different types of renal scans, and they can be used to check the kidneys along with other imaging methods such as ultrasound, CT scans, and MRIs. Sometimes they can provide unique information that is hard to get from other imaging procedures. A health-care professional determines which method will provide the best information about your kidneys and urinary system.

- **Positron emission tomography (PET).** A PET scan is a type of imaging that uses a small amount of radioactive material, a special camera, and a computer to help health-care professionals see how the organs and tissues are working. PET scans are sometimes performed on combined PET/CT scanners.

HOW DO YOU PREPARE FOR AN IMAGING TEST?

How you prepare for an imaging test will depend on the test's purpose and type. Your health-care professional will give you instructions. Listen carefully and ask questions if you do not understand. Before undergoing certain imaging tests, you might be asked to prepare in specific ways:

- Drink several glasses of water two hours before some ultrasound tests.
- Take a laxative for a transrectal ultrasound.
- Take an enema about four hours before a transrectal ultrasound.
- Talk with the technical staff about any implanted devices that may have metal parts, such as heart pacemakers, intrauterine devices (IUDs), hip replacements, implanted ports for catheters, and metallic items, such as metal plates, pins, screws, surgical staples, bullets, or shrapnel.
- Take a sedative before an MRI or CT scan if you feel anxious or have difficulty holding still in enclosed spaces.
- Discuss with your health-care professional if there is any chance you may be pregnant and whether the imaging uses x-rays.
- Fast for 12 hours before the test.

WHAT HAPPENS AFTER YOUR IMAGING TEST?

After most imaging tests, you can go home and resume normal activity. Some tests that involve catheters may cause minor discomfort. Tests that include medication, dyes, or sedatives occasionally trigger allergic reactions.

Tests that may cause discomfort include the following:

- **Tests involving a catheter in the urethra**. You might feel some mild discomfort from an irritated urethra for a few hours after the procedure.
- **Transrectal ultrasound**. You might feel some discomfort from an irritated rectum.

If you have a catheterization, your health-care professional may prescribe an antibiotic for one or two days to prevent an infection. If you have any signs of infection, including pain, chills, or fever, call your health-care professional immediately.

Tests that may cause an allergic reaction include the following:

- **Tests involving contrast medium**. If you have a rare sign of reaction, such as hives, itching, nausea, vomiting, headache, or dizziness, call your health-care professional immediately.
- **Tests involving sedatives**. If you have a rare sign of a reaction, such as changes in breathing and heart rate, call your health-care professional immediately.

HOW SOON WILL TEST RESULTS BE AVAILABLE?

For simple tests, such as x-rays and abdominal ultrasounds, you can discuss the results with your health-care professional soon afterward. Results of other tests, such as MRIs or CT scans, may take several days to become available, and you may need a separate appointment to discuss your results.[1]

Section 30.2 | **Kidney Biopsy**

WHAT IS A KIDNEY BIOPSY?

A kidney biopsy is a procedure in which a health-care professional takes one or more tiny pieces of tissue from your kidney. A pathologist

[1] "Urinary Tract Imaging," National Institute of Diabetes and Digestive and Kidney Diseases (NIDDK), April 2020. Available online. URL: www.niddk.nih.gov/health-information/diagnostic-tests/urinary-tract-imaging. Accessed October 25, 2024.

examines the tissue samples under a microscope for signs of damage or disease.

WHY DO HEALTH-CARE PROFESSIONALS USE KIDNEY BIOPSY?

A kidney biopsy can help health-care professionals diagnose and treat kidney problems when they need more information after looking at your blood and urine tests. A biopsy may be recommended if your lab test results show any of these conditions:

- persistent blood in your urine, known as "hematuria"
- too much protein in your urine, known as "proteinuria"
- problems with kidney function, which can cause waste products to build up in your blood

A kidney biopsy can help health-care professionals:

- check for signs of kidney inflammation, scarring, infection, or unusual deposits of a protein called "immunoglobulin"
- identify which parts of your kidney are damaged and how likely it is the damage will get worse
- determine the best way to treat your kidney problem

If you have a transplanted kidney that is not working properly, the biopsy can help your health-care professional find the cause.

In some cases, a kidney biopsy may be used to examine an abnormal mass or lump seen on a kidney x-ray or ultrasound and help rule out kidney cancer.

HOW DO I PREPARE FOR A KIDNEY BIOPSY?

Talk with Your Health-Care Professional

Talk with your health-care professional about what you can expect before, during, and after the kidney biopsy. If you have high blood pressure, your health-care professional may discuss ways to control it before the procedure. High blood pressure that is not well controlled by medicines can increase the risk of bleeding after a kidney biopsy.

Some medicines and supplements can increase the risk of bleeding or affect how you respond to sedatives or anesthesia. Review with your health-care professional all your prescribed and over-the-counter medicines, vitamins, and supplements, including:

- aspirin
- nonsteroidal anti-inflammatory drugs (NSAIDs)
- blood thinners

Tell your health-care professional about any allergies you have to medicines or foods.

Follow Your Health-Care Professional's Instructions

- Make any needed changes to the medicines and supplements you take.
- Have blood tests and imaging tests—such as a computed tomography (CT) scan or ultrasound—to prepare for the procedure.
- Make plans to get a ride home after the kidney biopsy.
- Fast for several hours before the procedure.
- Arrive 90 minutes to two hours before the procedure to sign a consent form and have any needed tests.

HOW DO HEALTH-CARE PROFESSIONALS PERFORM A KIDNEY BIOPSY?

The kidney biopsy is usually performed by a radiologist or nephrologist at a hospital or outpatient center.

Percutaneous Kidney Biopsy

A health-care professional inserts a thin biopsy needle through your skin and into your kidney to obtain samples of your kidney tissue for analysis. Most kidney biopsies are done this way.

The procedure usually takes about an hour. In most cases, you will lie face down with a firm pillow or sandbag under your body. If you have a transplanted kidney, you will lie on your back because health-care professionals place transplanted kidneys in the front lower part of the abdomen. If you are pregnant or have severe obesity, the procedure may sometimes be done while you are lying down, seated, or in another position that is comfortable for you.

A health-care professional may give you an intravenous (IV) sedative through a line placed in a vein in your arm or hand before the biopsy. The sedative will help you stay comfortable during the procedure. After marking the spot where the needle will enter your skin, a health-care professional will clean the area and inject a local anesthetic to numb the area.

Next, a health-care professional will use imaging methods—most often, an ultrasound—to guide the biopsy needle. The health-care professional may insert the needle more than once to obtain enough tissue for a diagnosis. The needle often has a trigger to ensure it goes in and out of the kidney quickly, and it can make a clicking or popping sound, which is normal. The health-care professional may ask you to hold your breath for a few moments during the biopsy.

After the biopsy, no stitches are needed. A health-care professional will place a bandage over the spot where the needle entered your skin.

Other Methods

If a percutaneous kidney biopsy is not a good option for you, your health-care professional may recommend one of the following procedures:

- **Laparoscopic kidney biopsy**. A health-care professional makes two small cuts into your back and inserts special tools to view your kidney and collect tissue samples. The procedure is done while you are under general anesthesia.
- **Transjugular kidney biopsy**. A health-care professional inserts a catheter and needle into a vein in your neck called the "jugular vein." The biopsy needle is guided through your veins and into your kidney to collect a tissue sample. This method of obtaining kidney tissue is used less often than the laparoscopic method.
- **Open kidney biopsy**. A health-care professional makes a small cut in your skin close to your kidney, takes a

small tissue sample, and stitches the cut closed. This procedure requires general anesthesia and is used rarely.

WHAT SHOULD I EXPECT AFTER A KIDNEY BIOPSY?

Recovery

After a kidney biopsy, you should expect the following:

- **Lie down in a recovery room for several hours while your blood pressure, pulse, and urine are monitored.** A health-care professional will also check to ensure there is no internal bleeding at the biopsy site.
- **Be released to rest at home.** In some cases, you may need to stay overnight at the hospital.
- **You may experience pain or soreness near the biopsy site.** You may also pass pink or slightly cloudy urine for up to 24–48 hours after the procedure.
- **Wait two weeks before resuming strenuous activities, such as heavy lifting or participating in contact sports.**

Biopsy Results

After the biopsy, your kidney tissue will be sent to a lab to be examined by a pathologist. Biopsy results may take a few days or longer to come back. In urgent cases, your health-care professional may receive a preliminary report within 24 hours. Your health-care professional will review the results with you during a follow-up visit.

WHAT ARE THE RISKS OF A KIDNEY BIOPSY?

The risks of a kidney biopsy include:

- bleeding from the biopsy site (A small amount of bleeding is common after a kidney biopsy. The bleeding is rarely serious enough to require treatment or a blood transfusion. Bleeding that is serious enough to require surgery or cause the loss of a kidney is very rare.)
- pain at the biopsy site, which is usually mild and goes away a few hours after the procedure
- infection, which is rare

Seek Care Right Away

Seek medical help immediately if you have any of these symptoms after a kidney biopsy:

- cannot urinate, have to urinate very often, feel the urge to go to the bathroom right away, or have a burning feeling when urinating
- have urine that is dark red or brown or has blood clots
- feel worsening pain at the biopsy site
- see redness, swelling, bleeding, or other drainage from the biopsy site
- have a fever
- feel faint or dizzy[1]

[1] "Kidney Biopsy," National Institute of Diabetes and Digestive and Kidney Diseases (NIDDK), March 2022. Available online. URL: www.niddk.nih.gov/health-information/diagnostic-tests/kidney-biopsy. Accessed October 25, 2024.

Part 6 | Kidney Failure: End-Stage Renal Disease

Chapter 31 | Managing Life with Kidney Failure

UNDERSTANDING KIDNEY FAILURE

If your kidney function drops below 15 percent of normal, you are said to have kidney failure. You may have symptoms from the buildup of waste products and extra water in your body.

To replace your lost kidney function, you may have one of three treatment options:

- hemodialysis
- peritoneal dialysis
- kidney transplant

End-stage renal disease (ESRD) is kidney failure that is treated by dialysis or kidney transplant.

Some people with kidney failure choose not to have dialysis or a transplant but continue to receive care from their health-care team, take medicines, and monitor their diet and lifestyle choices.

Work with your health-care team and family to consider your options and choose a treatment that is right for you. Treatment will help you feel better and live longer.

The more you know ahead of time about what to expect, the better prepared you may be to make a treatment choice and take charge of your care. You also need to give yourself time to get used to the big changes that will be happening in your life. Kidney failure will change your day-to-day activities, relationships with friends and family, and how you feel.

SYMPTOMS OF KIDNEY FAILURE

Symptoms of kidney failure may begin so slowly that you do not notice them right away.

Healthy kidneys prevent the buildup of wastes and extra fluid in your body and balance the salts and minerals in your blood—such as calcium, phosphorus, sodium, and potassium. Your kidneys also make hormones that help control blood pressure, make red blood cells, and keep your bones strong.

Kidney failure means your kidneys no longer work well enough to do these jobs and, as a result, other health problems develop. As your kidney function goes down, you may:

- have swelling, usually in your legs, feet, or ankles
- get headaches
- feel itchy
- feel tired during the day and have sleep problems at night
- feel sick to your stomach, lose your sense of taste, not feel hungry, or lose weight
- make little or no urine
- have muscle cramps, weakness, or numbness
- have pain, stiffness, or fluid in your joints
- feel confused, have trouble focusing, or have memory problems

Following your treatment plan can help you avoid or address most of these symptoms. Your treatment plan may include regular dialysis treatments or a kidney transplant, a special eating plan, physical activity, and medicines.

LIVING WELL WITH KIDNEY FAILURE

Doing well with kidney failure is a challenge. You will feel better if you:

- stick to your treatment schedule
- review your medicines with your health-care provider at every visit and take your medicines as prescribed
- work with a dietitian to develop an eating plan that includes foods you enjoy eating while also helping your health

- stay active—take a walk or do some other physical activity that you enjoy
- stay in touch with your friends and family

Treatment with dialysis or transplant will help you feel better and live longer. Your health-care team will work with you to create a treatment plan to address any health problems you have. Your treatment will include steps you can take to maintain your quality of life and activity level.

Your eating plan plays an important role. When you have kidney failure, what you eat and drink may help you maintain a healthy balance of salts, minerals, and fluids in your body.

STAYING ACTIVE WITH KIDNEY FAILURE

Physical activity is an important part of staying healthy when you have kidney failure. Being active strengthens your muscles, bones, and heart. It also makes your blood travel through your body faster, allowing your body to get more oxygen. Your body needs oxygen to use the energy from food.

You may find that physical activity can also improve your mood and make you feel better.

Talk with your doctor before you start a new exercise routine. Start slowly, with easier activities such as walking at a normal pace or gardening. Work up to harder activities such as walking briskly. Aim to be active on as many days as possible.

SLEEP AND KIDNEY FAILURE

People who have kidney failure may have trouble sleeping. Sleep loss can affect your quality of life, energy level, and mood. Restless leg syndrome, sleep apnea, pain, or itching may make it hard for you to sleep.

You can take several steps to improve your sleep habits. For example, physical activity during the day and a warm bath before bed may help you sleep better at night. Avoid caffeine after lunchtime, alcoholic drinks before bed, and smoking.

Talk with your health-care provider if you often feel sleepy during the day or have trouble sleeping at night. Health-care providers can treat sleep disorders such as sleep apnea or restless leg syndrome.

EFFECT ON SEXUAL LIFE

Kidney failure will affect your emotions, nerves, hormones, and energy levels, all of which may change your sexual relationships. Taking good care of yourself by managing your kidney disease and controlling your blood pressure and blood glucose levels can help prevent some sexual problems, such as erectile dysfunction. Getting counseling may help with some emotional problems, such as anxiety and depression, which can get in the way of having satisfying sex.

You may feel shy asking questions about your sex life, but your health-care team has heard the same questions from other people. Your provider is trained to help you address concerns about your sex life.

EMPLOYMENT WITH KIDNEY FAILURE

Many people with kidney failure continue to work. KidneyWorks is a program to help people with kidney disease keep working (https://kidneyworks.org/white-paper-and-executive-summary). The program focuses on Americans with chronic kidney disease (CKD) whose kidneys have not yet failed or who are living with a transplant. If you are on dialysis, the information in the KidneyWorks paper may also provide tips to help you keep your job.

The Americans with Disabilities Act (ADA; www.ada.gov) means that an employer cannot legally fire you just because you are on dialysis or have had a kidney transplant. The law requires an employer to make reasonable changes to the workplace for a person with a disability. For example, your employer may give you lighter physical jobs or schedule your work hours around your dialysis sessions. If you are on peritoneal dialysis, you will need space and time to change the dialysis solution in the middle of the workday. Most employers can make these adjustments.

If your employer is not willing to meet your needs, your dialysis clinic's renal social worker may be able to help find a way to satisfy both you and your employer.

EMOTIONAL WELL-BEING WITH KIDNEY FAILURE

Coping with kidney failure can be stressful. Some of the steps that you are taking to manage your kidney disease are also healthy ways to cope with stress. For example, physical activity and sleep help reduce stress. Learn more about healthy ways to cope with stress.

Depression is common among people with a chronic, or long-term, illness. Depression can make it harder to manage your kidney disease. Ask for help if you feel down. Your health-care team can help you. Talking with a support group, clergy member, friend, or family member who will listen to your feelings may help. Treatment for depression is available.

TAKING CHARGE OF YOUR MEDICAL CARE

Taking charge of your own medical care can help you feel more in control of your life. Take all your medicines and keep all your appointments. Work with your health-care team to learn about different kidney failure treatments, and let them know what kind of treatment you want. Ask questions when your health-care provider tells you something you do not understand. If you choose home hemodialysis or peritoneal dialysis, tell your dialysis nurse about any problems you have with equipment or supplies. If you have a transplant, talk with your transplant coordinator if your medicines cause side effects. You are your own best advocate.[1]

[1] "What Is Kidney Failure?" National Institute of Diabetes and Digestive and Kidney Diseases (NIDDK), January 2018. Available online. URL: www.niddk.nih.gov/health-information/kidney-disease/kidney-failure/what-is-kidney-failure. Accessed October 25, 2024.

Chapter 32 | End-Stage Renal Disease in Children

End-stage renal disease (ESRD) is a medical condition in which a person's kidneys cease functioning on a permanent basis, leading to the need for a regular course of long-term dialysis or a kidney transplant to maintain life.

TRENDS IN END-STAGE RENAL DISEASE INCIDENCE AND PREVALENCE

From 2011 to 2021, the adjusted incidence of ESRD in children decreased by about 10 percent, whereas the adjusted prevalence of ESRD increased by 1.8 percent. This suggests that children with ESRD may be surviving longer than in the past (or perhaps being diagnosed at a younger age as they do "age out" of the group at age 18). Indeed, first-year mortality has decreased over time, at least prior to a recent increase in the coronavirus 2019 (COVID-19) era. Consistent with this, the prevalence of children with a functioning kidney transplant increased by approximately 6 percent over the decade, and, as of 2021, over three-quarters of children with ESRD had a functioning kidney transplant.

RACIAL AND ETHNIC DISPARITIES IN END-STAGE RENAL DISEASE INCIDENCE

There are substantial differences in ESRD incidence by race and ethnicity among children. Although incidence can vary significantly by year, especially in smaller groups such as Asian children, the adjusted incidence of ESRD in 2021 was one-and-a-half times as high in Black children as in white children and was twice as high in Black children as in Asian children. As a result, there were also large differences in the prevalence of ESRD by race and ethnicity.

Treatment Disparities

The treatment of ESRD also differed by race and ethnicity: a much higher percentage of Black (56%) and Hispanic (53%) children initiated hemodialysis (HD) as the first treatment modality for kidney failure compared with white (36%) children. Differences in ESRD treatment by race may be due to the epidemiology of kidney disease: younger children with ESRD due to congenital anomalies of the kidney and urinary tract (CAKUT) are relatively more likely to be white (and, because they are young, to receive peritoneal dialysis (PD) or a transplant), whereas older children with ESRD due to glomerulonephritis are relatively more likely to be Black and, as a result, to be treated with HD. The rate of receipt of a kidney transplant among white children receiving dialysis was double that of Black and Hispanic children, and the pattern was similar for preemptive transplantation.

CHANGES IN WAITLISTING FOR KIDNEY TRANSPLANT

Although the percentage of children who were waitlisted for a kidney transplant prior to initiating dialysis nearly doubled between 2011 and 2021, the percentage of children who were waitlisted or transplanted within the year after ESRD onset, which had been relatively stable at around 50 percent from 2011 to 2020, decreased abruptly in 2021 to approximately 41 percent. The reasons for this decrease are unclear, but it may represent a lagging effect of the pandemic (e.g., delays in evaluating potential living donors in 2020).

TIME ON THE WAITLIST AND OUTCOMES

The median time on the waitlist for a kidney-alone transplant among children remained relatively unchanged, at approximately six months, between 2011 and 2021. Whether it increased in 2022 will be reported in the 2024 Annual Data Report. As with other aspects of pediatric ESRD care, outcomes varied by race: the time to 50 percent incidence of kidney transplant among children treated with dialysis was substantially longer for Black children (28.5 months) than for white children (18.6 months), and the transplant rate in Black children was substantially lower.

HOSPITALIZATION BURDEN

Hospitalization imposes a substantial burden on children. In the year after ESRD onset, children spent an average of approximately 13 days in the hospital, with children receiving PD and young children (those aged <6 years) being disproportionately affected. Nonsurgical causes of hospitalization were far more common than surgical causes. Hospitalizations decreased from 2019 to 2021; however, this trend may reflect a general decline in hospitalizations across society.

Hospitalizations for infection in the year after ESRD onset decreased from 2006–2010 to 2016–2020 for children receiving dialysis, but strikingly did not decrease for children treated with a kidney transplant, who instead experienced an increase in infection-related hospitalizations. Indeed, in 2016–2020, rates of hospitalization differed little by ESRD treatment modality. The rate of hospitalization for COVID-19 infection, a subset of hospitalization for infection, was nearly double in Black compared with the rate in white children and was higher in children receiving HD than in children receiving PD or with a kidney transplant, suggesting that the in-center dialysis facility could have served as a locus of transmission.

OVERALL OUTCOMES

Overall, outcomes appear to have improved in children, at least prior to the onset of the pandemic: adjusted mortality in the first year of ESRD treatment was halved from 2004–2006 to 2016–2018, although it increased by 28 percent in 2019–2021.[1]

[1] "ESRD among Children and Adolescents," National Institute of Diabetes and Digestive and Kidney Diseases (NIDDK), November 2, 2023. Available online. URL: https://usrds-adr.niddk.nih.gov/2023/end-stage-renal-disease/8-esrd-among-children-and-adolescents. Accessed October 22, 2024.

Chapter 33 | Hemodialysis

WHAT IS HEMODIALYSIS?

Hemodialysis is a treatment to filter wastes and water from your blood, as your kidneys did when they were healthy. Hemodialysis helps control blood pressure and balance important minerals, such as potassium, sodium, and calcium, in your blood.

Hemodialysis can help you feel better and live longer, but it is not a cure for kidney failure.

WHAT HAPPENS DURING HEMODIALYSIS?

During hemodialysis, blood passes through a filter called a "dialyzer" outside the body. A dialyzer is sometimes called an "artificial kidney."

At the start of a hemodialysis treatment, a dialysis nurse or technician places two needles into your arm. You may prefer to put in your own needles after you are trained by your health-care team. A numbing cream or spray can be used if placing the needles bothers you. Each needle is attached to a soft tube connected to the dialysis machine (see Figure 33.1).

The dialysis machine pumps blood through the filter and returns the blood to your body. During the process, the dialysis machine checks your blood pressure and controls how quickly:

- blood flows through the filter
- fluid is removed from your body

WHAT HAPPENS TO MY BLOOD WHILE IT IS IN THE FILTER?

Blood enters at one end of the filter and is forced into many very thin, hollow fibers. As your blood passes through the hollow fibers, the dialysis solution passes in the opposite direction on the outside of the fibers. Waste products from your blood move into the dialysis solution. Filtered blood remains in the hollow fibers and returns to your body.

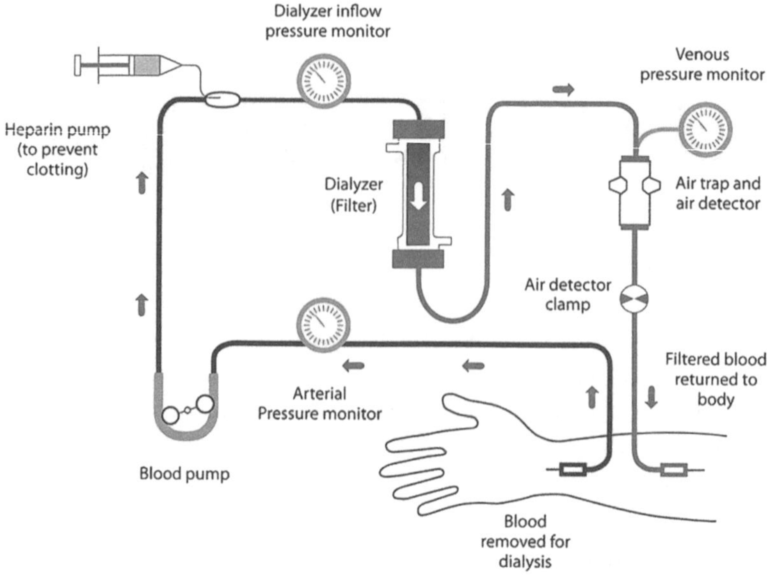

Figure 33.1. Hemodialysis

National Institute of Diabetes and Digestive and Kidney Diseases (NIDDK)

WHERE CAN I HAVE HEMODIALYSIS?

You can receive treatment at a dialysis center or at home. Each location has its pros and cons.

Dialysis Center

Most people go to a dialysis center for treatment. At the dialysis center, health-care professionals set up and help you connect to the dialysis machine. A team of health-care workers will be available to help you. You will continue to see your doctor. Other team members may include nurses, health-care technicians, a dietitian, and a social worker.

Home Hemodialysis

Home hemodialysis lets you have longer or more frequent dialysis, which comes closer to replacing the work healthy kidneys do—usually three to seven times per week, and with treatment sessions that last between 2 and 10 hours. Machines for home use are small enough to sit on an end table.

If you choose to have your treatments at home, you will still see your doctor once per month.

HOW DO I PREPARE FOR A HEMODIALYSIS?

Dialysis is a complex treatment that takes time to understand. Because most people do not feel sick until shortly before starting dialysis, you will likely still feel well when your doctor first talks to you about getting ready for dialysis. No one wants to start you on dialysis before you need it, but it takes time to prepare for dialysis.

Take Care of the Blood Vessels in Your Arms

It is important to protect the veins in your arm prior to starting dialysis. If you have kidney disease, remind health-care providers to draw blood and insert IV lines only in veins below your wrist; for example, ask them to use a vein in the back of your hand. If an arm vein is damaged by an IV line or by repeated blood draws, that vein may not be able to be used for dialysis.

Vascular Access Surgery

One important step before starting hemodialysis treatment is having minor surgery to create vascular access. Your vascular access will be your lifeline through which you will connect to the dialyzer. Dialysis moves blood through the filter at a high rate, and blood flow is very strong. The machine withdraws and returns almost a pint of blood to your body every minute. The access will be the place on your body where you insert needles to allow your blood to flow from and return to your body at a high rate during dialysis.

Three types of vascular access exist:

1. an arteriovenous (AV) fistula
2. an AV graft
3. a catheter

Work closely with your nephrologist and vascular surgeon—a surgeon who works with blood vessels—to make sure the access is in place in plenty of time. Healing may take several months. The goal is for your access to be ready for use when you are ready for dialysis.

WHAT CHANGES WILL I HAVE TO MAKE WHEN I START HEMODIALYSIS?

You have to adjust your life to build your dialysis treatment sessions into your routine. If you have in-center dialysis, you may need to rest after each treatment. Adjusting to the effects of kidney failure and the time you spend on dialysis can be hard. You may need to make changes in your work or home life, giving up some activities and responsibilities. Accepting these changes can be hard on you and your family. A mental health counselor or social worker can answer your questions and help you cope.

You will have to change what you eat and drink, and your health-care team may adjust the medicines you take.

HOW WILL I KNOW IF MY HEMODIALYSIS IS WORKING?

You will know your hemodialysis treatments are working by how you feel. Your energy level may increase, and you may have a better appetite. Hemodialysis reduces salt and fluid buildup, so you should also have less shortness of breath and swelling.

To make the most of your hemodialysis treatment, keep to your ideal "dry weight." Your ideal dry weight is your weight when you do not have extra fluid in your body. If you are careful about the sodium in your diet and the hemodialysis is working, you should be able to reach your ideal dry weight at the end of every hemodialysis treatment. When hemodialysis treatments are working, and you keep to your ideal dry weight, your blood pressure should be well controlled. In addition, blood tests can show how well your hemodialysis treatments are working. Once a month, whether you are on home or dialysis center hemodialysis, your dialysis center will test your blood. Read more about hemodialysis dose and adequacy.

WHAT ARE POSSIBLE PROBLEMS OF HEMODIALYSIS?

You could have a problem with your vascular access, which is the most common reason someone on hemodialysis needs to go to the hospital. Any type of vascular access may:

- become infected
- have poor blood flow or blockage from a blood clot or scar

These problems can prevent your treatments from working. For them to work properly, you may need more procedures to replace or repair your access.

Sudden changes in your body's water and chemical balance during treatment can cause additional problems, such as:

- muscle cramps
- a sudden drop in blood pressure, called "hypotension." Hypotension can make you feel weak, dizzy, or sick to your stomach.

Your doctor can change your dialysis solution to help avoid these problems. The longer and more frequent treatments of home hemodialysis are less likely to cause muscle cramps or rapid changes in blood pressure than standard in-center dialysis.

You can lose blood if a needle comes out of your access or a tube comes out of the dialyzer. To prevent blood loss, dialysis machines have a blood leak detector that sets off an alarm. If this problem occurs at the clinic, a nurse or technician will be on hand to act. If you are using home dialysis, your training will prepare you and your partner to fix the problem.

You may need a few months to adjust to hemodialysis. Always report problems to your health-care team, who often can treat side effects quickly and easily. You can avoid many side effects by following an eating plan you develop with your dietitian, limiting liquid intake, and taking your medicines as directed.

WHAT HAPPENS IF I HAVE BEEN ON DIALYSIS AND I DECIDE TO STOP?

If you have been on dialysis and wish to stop, you will still receive supportive care. The dialysis social worker may be able to help you develop an end-of-life care plan before you stop dialysis.[1]

[1] "Hemodialysis," National Institute of Diabetes and Digestive and Kidney Diseases (NIDDK), January 2018. Available online. URL: www.niddk.nih.gov/health-information/kidney-disease/kidney-failure/hemodialysis. Accessed October 20, 2024.

Chapter 34 | Peritoneal Dialysis

WHAT IS PERITONEAL DIALYSIS, AND HOW DOES IT WORK?

Peritoneal dialysis is a treatment for kidney failure that uses the lining of the abdomen, or belly, to filter blood inside the body. Health-care providers call this lining the peritoneum.

A few weeks before you start peritoneal dialysis, a surgeon places a soft tube, called a "catheter," in your belly.

When you start treatment, the dialysis solution—water with salt and other additives—flows from a bag through the catheter into your belly. When the bag is empty, you disconnect it and place a cap on your catheter so you can move around and do your normal activities. While the dialysis solution is inside your belly, it absorbs wastes and extra fluid from your body (see Figure 34.1).

After a few hours, the solution and waste are drained out of your belly into the empty bag. You can throw away the used solution in a toilet or tub. Then, you start over with a fresh bag of dialysis solution. When the solution is fresh, it absorbs wastes quickly. As time passes, filtering slows. For this reason, you need to repeat the process of emptying the used solution and refilling your belly with fresh solution four to six times every day. This process is called an "exchange."

You can do your exchanges during the day or at night using a machine that pumps the fluid in and out. For the best results, it is important that you perform all of your exchanges as prescribed. Dialysis can help you feel better and live longer, but it is not a cure for kidney failure.

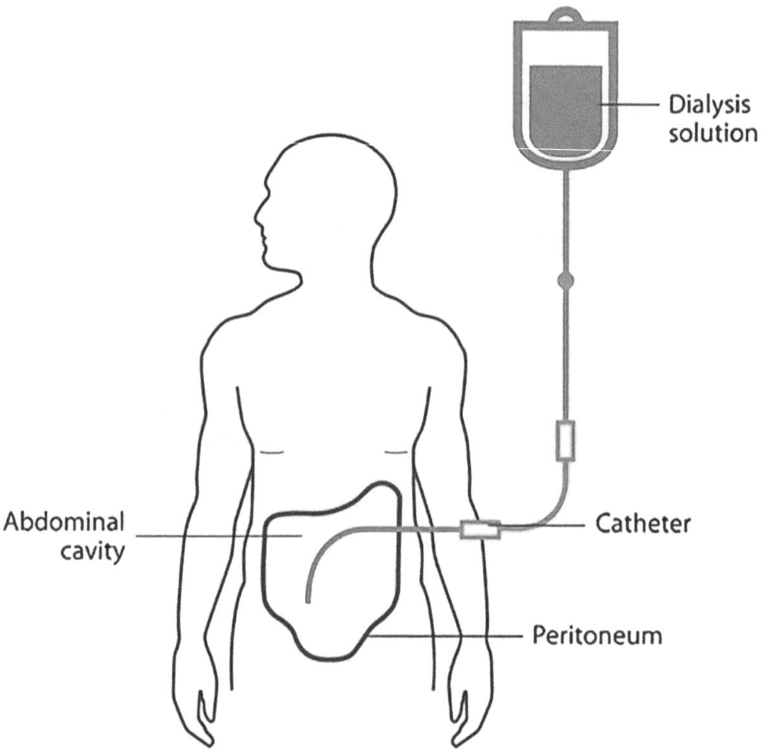

Figure 34.1. Peritoneal Dialysis

National Institute of Diabetes and Digestive and Kidney Diseases (NIDDK)

WHAT ARE THE TYPES OF PERITONEAL DIALYSIS?

You can choose the type of peritoneal dialysis that best fits your life:

- **Continuous ambulatory peritoneal dialysis (CAPD).** CAPD does not use a machine. You perform the exchanges manually during the day.
- **Automated peritoneal dialysis.** A machine performs the exchanges while you sleep.

The main differences between the two types of peritoneal dialysis are:

- the schedule of exchanges
- one uses a machine and the other is done by hand

If one type of peritoneal dialysis does not suit you, talk with your doctor about trying the other type.

WHERE CAN I DO PERITONEAL DIALYSIS?

You can do both CAPD and automated peritoneal dialysis in any clean, private place, including at home, at work, or when traveling.

Before you travel, you can have the manufacturer ship the supplies to where you are going so they will be there when you arrive. If you use automated peritoneal dialysis, you will have to carry your machine with you or plan to do exchanges by hand while you are away from home.

HOW DO I PREPARE FOR A PERITONEAL DIALYSIS?

Surgery to Place Your Catheter

Before your first treatment, you will have surgery to place a catheter into your belly. Planning your catheter placement at least three weeks before your first exchange can improve treatment success.

Although the catheter can be used for dialysis as soon as it is in place, it tends to work better when you have 10–20 days to heal before starting a full schedule of exchanges.

Your surgeon will make a small cut, often below and a little to the side of your belly button, and then guide the catheter through the slit into your peritoneal cavity. You will receive general or local anesthesia, and you may need to stay overnight in the hospital. However, most people can go home after the procedure.

Dialysis Training

After training, most people can perform both types of peritoneal dialysis on their own. You will work with a dialysis nurse for 1–2 weeks to learn how to do exchanges and avoid infections. Most people bring a family member or friend to training. With a trained friend or family member, you will be prepared in case you have a sick day and need help with exchanges.

If you choose automated peritoneal dialysis, you will learn how to:

- prepare the cycler
- connect the bags of dialysis solution
- place the drain tube

If you choose automated peritoneal dialysis, you also need to learn how to do exchanges by hand in case of a power failure or if you need an exchange during the day in addition to nighttime automated peritoneal dialysis.

HOW DO I PERFORM AN EXCHANGE?

You will need the following supplies:

- transfer set
- dialysis solution
- supplies to keep your exit site clean

If you choose automated peritoneal dialysis, you will need a cycler.

Your health-care team will provide everything you need to begin peritoneal dialysis and help you arrange to have supplies such as dialysis solution and surgical masks delivered to your home, usually once a month. Careful handwashing and wearing a surgical mask over your nose and mouth while you connect your catheter to the transfer set can help prevent infection.

WHAT CHANGES WILL I HAVE TO MAKE WHEN I START PERITONEAL DIALYSIS?

Daily Routine

Your schedule will change as you work your dialysis exchanges into your routine. If you do CAPD during the day, you have some control over when you do the exchanges. However, you will still need to stop your normal activities and take about 30 minutes to perform an exchange. If you do automated peritoneal dialysis, you will have to set up your cycler every night.

Physical Activity

When your belly is full of dialysis solution, you may need to limit some physical activities. You may still be active and play sports, but you should discuss your activities with your health-care team.

Make Changes to What You Eat and Drink

If you are on peritoneal dialysis, you may need to limit:

- sodium
- phosphorus
- calories in your eating plan

You may also need to consider the following:

- Watch how much liquid you drink and eat. Your dietitian will help you determine how much liquid you need to consume each day.
- Add protein to your diet because peritoneal dialysis removes protein.
- Choose foods with the right amount of potassium.
- Take supplements made for people with kidney failure.

Eating the right foods can help you feel better while you are on peritoneal dialysis. Talk with your dialysis center's dietitian to find a meal plan that works for you.

Medicines

Your doctor may make changes to the medicines you take.

Coping

Adjusting to the effects of kidney failure and the time you spend on dialysis can be hard for both you and your family. You may:

- have less energy
- need to give up some activities and duties at work or at home

A counselor or social worker can answer your questions and help you cope.

Take Care of Your Exit Site, Supplies, and Catheter to Prevent Infections

Your health-care team will show you how to keep your catheter clean to prevent infections. Here are some general rules:

- Store your supplies in a cool, clean, dry place.
- Inspect each bag of solution for signs of contamination, such as cloudiness, before you use it.

- Find a clean, dry, well-lit space to perform your exchanges.
- Wash your hands every time you need to handle your catheter.
- Clean your skin where your catheter enters your body every day, as instructed by your health-care team.
- Wear a surgical mask when performing exchanges.

WHAT ARE THE POSSIBLE PROBLEMS OF PERITONEAL DIALYSIS?

Possible problems from peritoneal dialysis include infection, hernia (area of weakness in your abdominal muscle), and weight gain.

HOW WILL I KNOW IF MY PERITONEAL DIALYSIS IS WORKING?

To find out if your dialysis exchanges are removing enough waste, you will have a blood test and collect used dialysis solution once a month. If you are still urinating, you may need to collect urine.

These tests help your doctor prescribe a dialysis schedule and dose to meet your health needs. If your dialysis schedule is not removing enough waste or your body is absorbing too much dextrose, your doctor will make adjustments.[1]

[1] "Peritoneal Dialysis," National Institute of Diabetes and Digestive and Kidney Diseases (NIDDK), January 2018. Available online. URL: www.niddk.nih.gov/health-information/kidney-disease/kidney-failure/peritoneal-dialysis. Accessed October 20, 2024.

Chapter 35 | Water Use and Management in Dialysis

During an average week of hemodialysis, a patient can be exposed to 300–600 liters of water, providing multiple opportunities for potential patient exposure to waterborne pathogens. Adverse patient outcomes, including outbreaks associated with water exposure in dialysis settings, have resulted from patient exposure to water via a variety of pathways, including improper formulation of dialysate with water containing high levels of chemical or biological contaminants, contamination of injectable medications with tap water, and reprocessing of dialyzers with contaminated water. For the health and safety of hemodialysis patients, it is vital to ensure the water used to perform dialysis is safe and clean.

ASSOCIATION FOR THE ADVANCEMENT OF MEDICAL INSTRUMENTATION WATER STANDARDS

The Association for the Advancement of Medical Instrumentation (AAMI), in conjunction with the International Standards Organization (ISO), has established chemical and microbiological standards for the water used to prepare dialysate, substitution fluid, or to reprocess hemodialyzers for renal replacement therapy. The AAMI standards address:

- equipment and processes used to purify water for the preparation of concentrates and dialysate, as well as the reprocessing of dialyzers for multiple uses
- the devices used to store and distribute this water
- the allowable and action threshold levels of water contaminants, bacterial cell counts, and endotoxins

BOIL WATER ADVISORY PROCEDURES

What Is a Boil Water Advisory?

A Boil Water Advisory (BWA) protects the community from waterborne infectious agents. It is issued only after careful consideration among representatives from public health, regulatory agencies, and municipal departments after positive tests (e.g., positive samples for fecal coliforms, changes in turbidity measurements) or line breaks.

Do Not Drink Water Advisory

Officials typically issue "do not drink water advisories" when tap water is, or could be, contaminated with harmful chemicals or toxins. Boiling water containing harmful chemicals or toxins does not make it safe to use.

Do not drink advisories may include information about preparing food or drinks, making ice, washing dishes, cleaning, brushing teeth, bathing, flushing toilets, and other activities.

CAN WE DIALYZE PATIENTS DURING A BOIL WATER ADVISORY?

Yes, if the water treatment components in use are sufficient to remove or destroy bacteria. Reverse Osmosis (RO) will protect the product water from microbial contamination. A Deionization (DI) unit does not remove or destroy bacteria, so if DI is being used as the main water treatment (rather than RO), you will need a submicron or endotoxin/ultrafilter downstream of the DI unit. If an ultraviolet (UV) irradiator is used, the filter should be located after the UV irradiator. Close monitoring of the resistivity of the product water will be needed to detect any decrease in quality. Also, consider weekly microbial assessment of the product water during the BWA.

Keep in close contact with the municipal water supplier. They may choose to "shock" treat (hyper chlorinate) their distribution system to bring it back into compliance with the acceptable standards for drinking water. If the city "shocks" its water system, you may see chlorine or chloramine breakthroughs. Review your testing procedures with staff and alert them to be vigilant for potential breakthroughs so that patients will be protected from exposure to chlorine or chloramine.[1]

[1] "Water Use in Dialysis," Centers for Disease Control and Prevention (CDC), March 26, 2024. Available online. URL: www.cdc.gov/dialysis-safety/hcp/recommendations-resources/water-use-in-dialysis.html. Accessed October 22, 2024.

Chapter 36 | **Kidney Transplantation**

Chapter Contents

UNDERSTANDING KIDNEY TRANSPLANTATION

Some people with kidney failure may be able to have a kidney transplant. During transplant surgery, a healthy kidney from a donor is placed into your body. The new donated kidney does the work that your two kidneys used to do.

A donated kidney can come from someone you do not know who has recently died (a deceased donor) or from a living person—a relative, spouse, or friend. Due to the shortage of kidneys, patients on the waiting list for a deceased donor kidney may wait many years.

A kidney transplant is a treatment for kidney failure; it is not a cure. You will need to take medicines every day to make sure your immune system does not reject the new kidney. You will also need to see your health-care professional regularly.

A working transplanted kidney does a better job of filtering wastes and keeping you healthy than dialysis. However, a kidney transplant is not for everyone. Your doctor may tell you that you are not healthy enough for transplant surgery.

TALK WITH YOUR DOCTOR

The first step is to talk with your doctor to find out whether you are a candidate for a transplant. If you are on dialysis, your dialysis team will also be part of the process. If you and your doctor think a kidney transplant is right for you, your doctor will refer you to a transplant center.

GET TESTED AT A TRANSPLANT CENTER

At the transplant center, you will meet members of your transplant team. You will have tests to make sure you are a good candidate for transplant.

Tests will include blood tests and tests to check your heart and other organs—to make sure you are healthy enough for surgery. Some conditions or illnesses could make a transplant less likely to succeed, such as cancer that is not in remission or current substance abuse.

You will also have tests to check your mental and emotional health. The transplant team must be sure you are prepared to care for a transplanted kidney. You will need to be able to understand and follow a schedule for taking the medicines you need after surgery.

In a process called "cross-matching," the transplant team tests the donor's blood against your blood to help predict whether your body's immune system will accept or reject the new kidney. A kidney from a relative is more likely to be a better tissue match than a kidney from someone who is not related to you.

If a family member or friend wants to donate a kidney and is a good match, that person will need a health exam to make sure he or she is healthy enough to be a donor. If you have a living donor, you do not need to be on a waiting list for a kidney and can schedule the surgery when it is best for you, your donor, and your surgeon.

Testing and evaluation at the transplant center may take several visits over weeks to months.

GET ON THE WAITING LIST

If your tests show you can have a transplant, your transplant center will add your name to the waiting list. Wait times can range from a few months to years. Most transplant centers give preference to people who have been on the waiting list the longest. Other factors, such as your age, where you live, and your blood type, may make your wait longer or shorter.

A transplant center can place you on the waiting list for a donor kidney if your kidney function is 20 or less—even if you are not on dialysis. While you wait for a kidney transplant, you may need to start dialysis.

HAVE MONTHLY BLOOD TESTS

While you wait for a kidney, you will need monthly blood tests. The center must have a recent sample of your blood to match with any kidney that becomes available.

HAVE YOUR KIDNEY TRANSPLANT

During kidney transplant surgery, a surgeon places a healthy kidney into your body. The surgery usually takes three or four hours. Surgeons usually transplant a kidney into the lower abdomen near the groin.

If a family member or friend is donating the kidney, you will schedule the surgery in advance. A kidney from a living donor does not have to be transported from one site to another, so it may be in better condition than a kidney from a deceased donor. Your surgical team will operate on you and your donor at the same time, usually in side-by-side rooms. One surgeon will remove the kidney from the donor, while another prepares you to receive the donated kidney.

Figure 36.1 illustrates how the transplanted kidney is connected to blood vessels and the bladder, enabling blood filtration and urine flow into the bladder via the ureter.

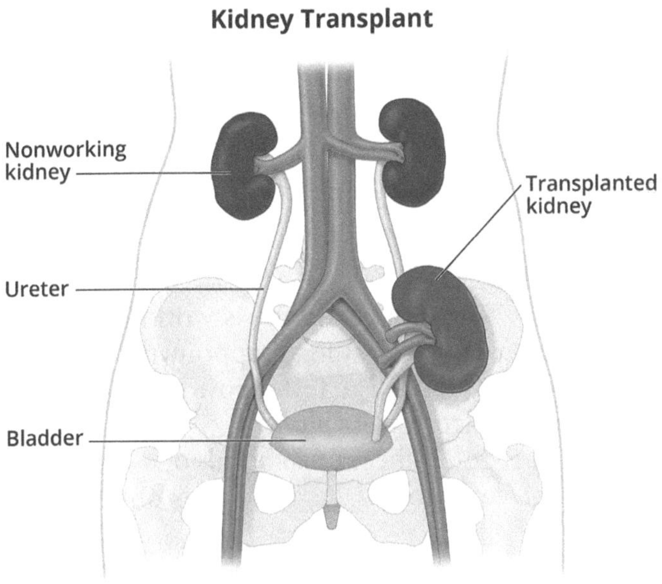

Figure 36.1. Kidney Transplant

National Institute of Diabetes and Digestive and Kidney Diseases (NIDDK)

RECOVERY AFTER YOUR TRANSPLANT

Many people report feeling much better right after having transplant surgery. For some people, it takes a few days for the new kidney to start working. You probably will need to stay in the hospital for several days to recover from surgery—longer if you have any problems after the transplant. You will have regular follow-up visits with your nephrologist after leaving the hospital.

If you have a living donor, the donor will probably also stay in the hospital for several days. However, a new technique for removing a kidney for donation that uses a smaller cut may allow the donor to leave the hospital in two to three days.

Before you leave the hospital, you need to learn how to stay healthy and take care of your donor kidney. You will have to take one or more anti-rejection medicines—also called "immunosuppressants." Without medicine, your immune system may treat your donor kidney as foreign, or not your own, and attack your new kidney. Anti-rejection medicines may have side effects.

You may also need to take other medicines—for example, antibiotics to protect against infections. Your transplant team will teach you what each medicine is for and when to take each one. Be sure you understand the instructions for taking your medicines before you leave the hospital.

MONITORING YOUR NEW KIDNEY

Blood tests help you know your donor kidney is working. Before you leave the hospital, you will schedule an appointment at the transplant center to test your blood. The tests show how well your kidneys are removing wastes from your blood.

At first, you will need regular checkups and blood tests at the transplant center or from your doctor. As time goes on, you will have fewer checkups.

Your blood tests may show that your kidney is not removing wastes from your blood as well as it should. You also may have other symptoms that your body is rejecting your donor kidney. If you have these problems, your transplant surgeon or nephrologist may order a kidney biopsy.

POSSIBLE PROBLEMS AFTER A KIDNEY TRANSPLANT

The donated kidney may start working right away or may take up to a few weeks to make urine. If the new kidney does not start working right away, you will need dialysis treatments to filter wastes and extra salt and fluid from your body until it starts working.

Other problems following the kidney transplant are similar to other pelvic surgeries and may include:

- bleeding
- infection, especially a bladder infection
- hernia
- pain or numbness along the inner thigh that usually goes away without treatment

Transplant rejection is rare right after surgery and can take days or weeks to occur. Rejection is less common when the new kidney is from a living donor than when it is from a deceased donor.

RECOGNIZING SYMPTOMS OF TRANSPLANT REJECTION

Transplant rejection often begins before you feel any changes. The routine blood tests that you have at the transplant center will reveal early signs of rejection. You may develop HBP or notice swelling because your kidney is not getting rid of extra salt and fluid in your body.

Your health-care provider will treat early signs of rejection by adjusting your medicines to help keep your body from rejecting your new kidney.

Transplant rejection is becoming less common. However, your body may still reject the donor kidney, even if you do everything you should. If that happens, you may need to go on dialysis and go back on the waiting list for another kidney. Some people are able to get a second kidney transplant.

Seek Medical Care Right Away

When you are taking anti-rejection medicines, you are at a greater risk for infection. Anti-rejection medicines can dull symptoms of problems such as infection. Call your transplant center right away if you are not feeling well or have:

- a fever of more than 100 degrees
- drainage from your surgical scar
- burning when you pass urine
- a cold or cough that will not go away

SIDE EFFECTS OF ANTI-REJECTION MEDICINES

Some anti-rejection medicines may change your appearance. Your face may get fuller, you may gain weight, or you may develop acne or facial hair. Not all people have these side effects.

Anti-rejection medicines weaken your immune system, which can lead to infections. In some people over long periods of time, a weakened immune system can increase their risk of developing cancer. Some anti-rejection medicines cause cataracts, diabetes, extra stomach acid, HBP, and bone disease.

When used over time, these medicines may also cause liver or kidney damage in some people. Your transplant team will order regular tests to monitor the levels of anti-rejection medicines in your blood and to measure your liver and kidney function.

DIETARY CONSIDERATIONS AFTER A KIDNEY TRANSPLANT

You have more choices about what to eat after you receive a kidney transplant than you would if you were on dialysis. However, you will need to work with a dietitian to develop an eating plan that can change in response to your medicines, test results, weight, and blood pressure.

FINANCIAL ASPECTS OF KIDNEY TRANSPLANTATION

Medicare, the federal government health insurance program, will pay for transplant and care for three years after the transplant. Medicare will also pay for your donor's surgery and his or her care. Medicare and private insurance may help pay for your medicines. Additionally, drug companies give discounts to people who can show that they cannot afford to pay for their prescriptions. Talk with your transplant social worker to find out what resources may be available to help you pay for your transplant.[1]

[1] "Kidney Transplant," National Institute of Diabetes and Digestive and Kidney Diseases (NIDDK), January 2018. Available online. URL: www.niddk.nih.gov/health-information/kidney-disease/kidney-failure/kidney-transplant. Accessed October 25, 2024.

Section 36.2 | Noninvasive Biomarkers for Kidney Transplant Rejection Detection

Levels of a protein in the urine of kidney transplant recipients can distinguish those at low risk of developing kidney injury from those at high risk, a study suggests. The results also suggest that low levels of this protein, called "CXCL9," can rule out rejection as a cause of kidney injury.

To prevent rejection, kidney transplant recipients typically take immunosuppressive drugs every day. However, these drugs can cause kidney damage and lead to other serious side effects, such as cancer, infection, and infertility. Even with immunosuppressive therapy, 10–15 percent of kidney recipients experience rejection during the first year after transplantation.

Currently, the only definitive way to distinguish rejection from other causes of kidney injury is by performing a biopsy, in which doctors remove a small piece of kidney tissue to look for rejection-associated damage. Although this procedure is generally considered safe, it carries some minor risks for the patient and does not always provide an accurate impression of the overall state of the kidney.

"A noninvasive urine test to accurately monitor the risk of kidney rejection could dramatically reduce the need for biopsies and possibly enable doctors to safely reduce immunosuppressive therapy in some patients," said National Institute of Allergy and Infectious Diseases (NIAID) Director Anthony S. Fauci, MD. "The results of this study support the further development of noninvasive tests for the detection and management of transplant rejection."

In this multicenter Clinical Trials in Organ Transplantation study, doctors periodically collected urine samples from 280 adult and child kidney transplant recipients for two years after transplantation. Investigators led by Peter Heeger, MD, of the Icahn School of Medicine at Mount Sinai in New York City, and Donald Hricik, MD, of Case Western Reserve University in Cleveland, measured the urinary levels of molecules that had previously been associated with rejection. These included two proteins and nine messenger RNAs (mRNAs)—intermediary molecules in the construction of proteins from genes. They identified CXCL9 protein and CXCL9 mRNA as potential biomarkers—molecules that indicate the effect or progress of a disease—for the diagnosis of rejection.

After further testing, the researchers found that CXCL9 protein was better at ruling out rejection than any of the mRNAs tested. Low levels of the protein biomarker also could identify patients likely to have stable long-term kidney function. Transplant recipients with low urinary CXCL9 protein six months after transplantation were unlikely to experience rejection or loss of kidney function over the next 18 months. In addition, the detection of the protein in the urine of transplant recipients was more straightforward than measuring mRNA levels. While proteins can be measured directly in urine, mRNAs must first be extracted from urine samples. The researchers obtained sufficient mRNA from just 76 percent of samples, highlighting the technical challenges of extraction.

"The relative ease of measuring urinary proteins suggests that developing a protein-based urine test for use in clinical practice would be less complicated than an mRNA test," said Daniel Rotrosen, MD, director of NIAID's Division of Allergy, Immunology, and Transplantation. "There is strong precedent for the development and use of tests that measure urinary proteins, such as home pregnancy tests."

CXCL9 protein levels also may be useful for predicting and monitoring transplant rejection. The investigators noted that urinary CXCL9 levels began to increase up to 30 days before clinical signs of kidney injury, which could allow doctors to intervene early to potentially avoid rejection-associated kidney damage. The protein levels began to drop after treatment for rejection, suggesting that the urine test could be used to monitor treatment progress.

"Development of noninvasive tests to detect immune activation before kidney damage occurs would help guide the care of kidney transplant recipients," said NIAID Transplantation Branch Chief Nancy Bridges, MD, a co-author of the paper. "Clinical application of the findings from this study could help avoid unnecessary biopsies and excess immunosuppression."[1]

---

[1] News and Events, "Protein-Based Urine Test Predicts Kidney Transplant Outcomes," National Institutes of Health (NIH), August 22, 2013. Available online. URL: www.nih.gov/news-events/news-releases/protein-based-urine-test-predicts-kidney-transplant-outcomes. Accessed October 25, 2024.

Chapter 37 | Conservative Management for Kidney Failure

WHAT IS CONSERVATIVE MANAGEMENT?

Conservative management for kidney failure means that your health-care team continues your care without dialysis or a kidney transplant. The focus of care is on your quality of life and symptom control.

You have the right to decide how your kidney failure will be treated. You can choose conservative management instead of dialysis or transplant.

You may hear conservative management referred to as "comprehensive conservative care," "supportive care," "nondialytic care," and "comfort care." You might also encounter the term "palliative care," which is one part of conservative management. Palliative care addresses the physical, psychological, and spiritual needs of someone with a serious illness.

WHAT HAPPENS IF I CHOOSE CONSERVATIVE MANAGEMENT?

Your health-care team will help you create a plan to meet your care needs. Your health-care team may include the following:

- nephrologist
- primary care clinician
- nurse
- dietitian
- social worker
- pharmacist

Treatment includes:

- preserving kidney function for as long as possible
- managing your symptoms, such as nausea, poor appetite, and emotional well-being
- managing other health problems caused by kidney failure, such as anemia
- maintaining your quality of life for as long as possible
- preparing for end-of-life care

Conservative management will not cure kidney disease. The treatment goals are to:

- provide the best quality of life
- avoid treatments and hospital stays that may worsen quality of life, which may mean fewer medical appointments, blood draws, and medications

Your care plan may change as your quality of life and health status change. As you near the end of your life, you may choose hospice care.

WHAT IS HOSPICE?

Hospice is a program of care and support for people at the end of life. A trained team of health professionals and caregivers provides symptom and pain relief as well as emotional and spiritual support. The hospice team also supports family caregivers.

With hospice care, you may choose to die at home or in a home-like hospice setting instead of in a hospital.

Medicare, the federal health insurance program, covers hospice care.

WHO CHOOSES CONSERVATIVE MANAGEMENT?

People who wish to focus their care on the quality of their life may choose conservative management.

For most people, dialysis may extend and improve quality of life. However, for others, this may not be true. Dialysis may not lengthen life for all people who have kidney failure and can feel like an added burden, especially for people who have other serious health problems. Dialysis may not prolong or improve the quality of life for people who:

- are elderly and frail
- have other serious health problems, such as dementia, heart failure, or cancer

Your health-care provider can help you and your family understand your health status so you can make an informed decision.

WHAT SHOULD I EAT WHILE ON CONSERVATIVE MANAGEMENT?

What you eat and drink may help you feel better and may help prolong your life. Work with a dietitian to help you choose what to eat.

HOW WILL I FEEL?

As waste products build up in your blood, your appetite may decline, and you may become less alert. Your health-care team can help you address these and other symptoms.

HOW LONG CAN I LIVE IF I CHOOSE CONSERVATIVE MANAGEMENT?

The answer to this question varies for each person. If you need dialysis to survive and do not receive it, you may live a few days or weeks.[1]

[1] "Conservative Management for Kidney Failure," National Institute of Diabetes and Digestive and Kidney Diseases (NIDDK), January 2018. Available online. URL: www.niddk.nih.gov/health-information/kidney-disease/kidney-failure/conservative-management. Accessed October 22, 2024.

Chapter 38 | Kidney Failure Treatment and Financial Assistance

Kidney failure treatment—hemodialysis, peritoneal dialysis, and kidney transplantation—is expensive. Many people with kidney failure need help paying for their care.

For many people with kidney failure, the federal government—through Medicare—helps pay for much of the cost of their treatment. The U.S. Congress passed the Social Security Amendments of 1972 that guarantee Medicare coverage for most people with kidney failure—even those under age 65.

You can also find financial help for kidney failure treatment from other sources, such as joint federal-state programs, private health insurance, private organizations, and medication assistance programs.

The amount you pay for premiums, copays, coinsurance, deductibles, prescriptions, and other costs is based on the services and medicines you need and the health-care coverage you have. You can live for years with kidney failure, so it is important that you get help to pay for your treatment.

FEDERAL GOVERNMENT HEALTH INSURANCE

What Is Medicare?

Medicare is a federal health insurance program that pays health-care costs for eligible people who are:

- age 65 or older
- under age 65 with certain disabilities and those who have received Social Security Disability Insurance (SSDI) for 2 years

- of any age with end-stage renal disease (ESRD)—permanent kidney failure treated with a kidney transplant or blood-filtering treatments called "dialysis"

What Health Plans Does Medicare Offer?

Medicare has two main ways to get coverage—Original Medicare, which includes Part A and B, or a Medicare Advantage Plan, also called "Part C." You can also choose to have prescription drug coverage through Medicare Part D.

Most people with kidney failure are not allowed to join a Medicare Advantage plan. However, beginning in 2021, the 21st Century Cures Act will allow people with ESRD to choose a Medicare Advantage plan instead of Original Medicare. Medicare Advantage plans may limit where you get care, but they cap out-of-pocket costs. With Original Medicare, there is no cap on out-of-pocket costs, but you can get care anywhere that Medicare is accepted.

When Does Medicare Coverage Start for People with End-Stage Renal Disease?

If kidney failure is the only reason you are signing up for Medicare, your Medicare start date will depend on the type of kidney failure treatment you receive.

When Does Medicare Coverage End for People with End-Stage Renal Disease?

If kidney failure is the only reason you have Medicare, your coverage end date will depend on whether you had a kidney transplant or dialysis treatment. Medicare coverage will not end if you are eligible because of age or disability.

JOINT FEDERAL-STATE PROGRAMS

You may also be able to get help paying for your kidney failure treatment from one or more programs run jointly by the federal and state governments, including Medicaid and the Children's Health Insurance Program (CHIP).

What Is Medicaid?

Medicaid provides free or low-cost health coverage for some low-income people, families and children, pregnant women, the elderly, and people with disabilities. Each state runs its own Medicaid program based on rules set by the federal government. Medicaid may pay for services that Medicare does not.

What Is the Children's Health Insurance Program?

The CHIP offers free or low-cost Medicaid to children whose parents earn too much for Medicaid but not enough to pay for a private health plan. Based on federal rules, CHIP is run by the states. In some states, it may cover pregnant women and their parents.

OTHER FEDERAL PROGRAMS

What Other Federal Programs Can Help?

The Social Security Administration can provide financial help through two programs—Social Security Disability Insurance (SSDI) and Supplemental Security Income (SSI).

- **SSDI pays a monthly amount to people who cannot work and have paid enough Social Security taxes.** If you have an illness or injury that Social Security believes will keep you out of work for at least a year, SSDI payments may be an option. There is a five-month waiting period before SSDI payments begin.
- **SSI pays a monthly amount to disabled children and adults who earn little and do not have many financial assets.** A person who gets SSI may be able to get food stamps and Medicaid, too.

OTHER STATE PROGRAMS

What Other State Programs Can Help?

- **Medicare Savings Programs are programs in which your state may pay your Medicare premiums, deductibles, and/or coinsurance if you have a low income and few assets.** How Medicaid works in U.S. territories varies.

- **State Health Insurance Assistance Programs (SHIPs) give local advice about health insurance to people who have Medicare or who are eligible for Medicare.** SHIP counselors can help you choose the best plan for your needs.
- **State kidney programs provide financial help and other services to people with kidney disease.** Talk with your dialysis or transplant clinic social worker or financial counselor to find out if your state has a kidney program.
- **State Pharmaceutical Assistance Programs (SPAPs) help pay for prescription medicines in certain states.**

PRIVATE HEALTH INSURANCE

What Types of Private Health Insurance Can Help?

Some people with kidney failure use private health insurance to help pay for their health care.

- **Group health insurance.** People buy this kind of health insurance through their employer, union, or a family member's employer or union. Group health plans pay for the first 30 months from the time you become eligible for Medicare for kidney failure. After that, a group plan can work with Medicare to help pay for costs that are not paid for by Medicare, such as copays, coinsurance, and deductibles. If you have or are eligible for group health insurance, you can contact the benefits administrator at the company or union that provides your insurance to find out what the plan covers and how it works with Medicare.
- **Individual health insurance.** People buy this coverage for themselves and their families. The Health Insurance Marketplace offers health insurance plans to people who are legally present in the United States and who do not have any other health insurance options. You cannot enroll in a Health Insurance Marketplace plan if you already have Medicare. Some people choose to keep their Marketplace plan instead of enrolling in Medicare. You may pay more for Medicare later if

you do not enroll in Medicare when you first become eligible. Insurance companies, agents, brokers, and online insurance stores are other ways to find and buy individual health insurance plans.

- **Medigap or Medicare Supplemental Insurance**. People buy this extra health insurance from a private company. Medigap plans help cover some costs that are not covered by Original Medicare, such as copays, coinsurance, and deductibles. If you are 65, federal law protects your right to buy a Medigap plan. If you are below 65 and are on dialysis, you may or may not be able to buy a Medigap policy from a licensed insurance company in your home state.[1]

[1] "Financial Help for Treatment of Kidney Failure," National Institute of Diabetes and Digestive and Kidney Diseases (NIDDK), February 1, 2020. Available online. URL: www.niddk.nih.gov/health-information/kidney-disease/kidney-failure/financial-help-treatment. Accessed October 25, 2024.

Chapter 39 | **Palliative and Hospice Care**

Palliative care and hospice care both focus on the comfort, care, and quality of life of individuals with a serious illness. Hospice care is a specific type of palliative care that is provided in the final weeks or months of life. Although these two forms of care are similar in some ways, they can differ regarding when and where care is received and which treatment options are available.

WHAT IS PALLIATIVE CARE?

Palliative care is focused on improving the quality of life for people with serious illnesses and their care partners. It is available to people of any age who need it, not just older adults. The major elements of palliative care include managing a person's symptoms effectively and ensuring that their care is coordinated.

Palliative care is interdisciplinary, meaning it involves multiple types of doctors and other care providers. These providers work together with patients and their families to ensure that the treatment plan reflects the person's goals and values.

Palliative care can start as early as a person's diagnosis or not until later in their illness, and it can occur alongside other types of treatment for the disease. This form of care includes but is not limited to, advance care planning, end-of-life care, hospice care, and bereavement support.

WHO CAN BENEFIT FROM PALLIATIVE CARE?

Palliative care is a resource for anyone living with a serious illness, such as heart failure, kidney failure, chronic obstructive pulmonary disease, cancer, dementia, Parkinson disease, and many others.

In addition to improving quality of life and helping with symptoms, palliative care can help patients understand their choices for medical treatment. The organized services available through palliative care may be helpful to any older person experiencing significant discomfort and disability later in life.

WHO MAKES UP THE PALLIATIVE CARE TEAM?

A palliative care team consists of multiple professionals who work with the patient, family, and the patient's other doctors to provide medical, social, emotional, and practical support. The team includes palliative care specialist doctors and nurses, as well as social workers, nutritionists, and chaplains. A person's team may vary based on their needs and level of care. To begin palliative care, a person's health-care provider may refer them to a palliative care specialist. If not suggested, the person can request a referral from their health-care provider.

WHERE IS PALLIATIVE CARE PROVIDED?

Palliative care can be provided in hospitals, nursing homes, outpatient palliative care clinics, certain specialized clinics, or at home. Medicare, Medicaid, and insurance policies may cover palliative care. Veterans may be eligible for palliative care through the Department of Veterans Affairs. Private health insurance might pay for some services. Health insurance providers can answer questions about coverage.

In palliative care, a person does not have to give up treatment that might cure a serious illness. Palliative care can be provided alongside curative treatment and may begin at the time of diagnosis. Over time, if the doctor or palliative care team believes ongoing treatment is no longer helping, there are two possibilities: palliative care could transition to hospice care if the doctor believes the person is likely to die within six months, or the palliative care team could continue to help with increasing emphasis on comfort care.

WHAT IS HOSPICE CARE?

Increasingly, people are choosing hospice care at the end of life. Hospice care focuses on the care, comfort, and quality of life of a person with a serious illness who is approaching the end of life.

At some point, it may not be possible to cure a serious illness, or a patient may choose not to undergo certain treatments. Hospice is designed for this situation. The patient beginning hospice care understands that their illness is not responding to medical attempts to cure it or slow the disease's progress.

Like palliative care, hospice provides comprehensive comfort care as well as support for the family, but in hospice, attempts to cure the person's illness are stopped. Hospice is provided for a person with a terminal illness whose doctor believes they have six months or less to live if the illness runs its natural course.

It is important for a patient to discuss hospice care options with their doctor. Sometimes, people do not begin hospice care soon enough to take full advantage of the help it offers. They may wait too long to begin hospice and find themselves too close to death. Some people are not eligible for hospice care soon enough to receive its full benefit. Starting hospice early may provide months of meaningful care and quality time with loved ones.

WHERE IS HOSPICE CARE PROVIDED, AND WHO PROVIDES IT?

Hospice is an approach to care, so it is not tied to a specific place. It can be offered in two types of settings: at home or in a facility such as a nursing home, hospital, or even a separate hospice center.

Hospice care brings together a team of people with special skills, including nurses, doctors, social workers, spiritual advisors, and trained volunteers. Everyone works together with the person who is dying, the caregiver, and/or the family to provide the medical, emotional, and spiritual support needed.

A member of the hospice team visits regularly, and someone is usually always available by phone—24 hours a day, 7 days a week. Hospice may be covered by Medicare and other insurance companies. It is advisable to check if insurance will cover the person's particular situation.

It is important to remember that stopping treatment aimed at curing an illness does not mean discontinuing all treatment. For example, if the doctor determines that cancer is not responding to chemotherapy and the patient chooses to enter hospice care, the chemotherapy will stop. Other medical care may continue as long as it is helpful. For example, if the person has high blood pressure, they will still receive medication for that condition.

Although hospice provides a lot of support, family and friends provide the day-to-day care of a person dying at home. The hospice team coaches family members on how to care for the dying person and even provides respite care when caregivers need a break. Respite care can last from a few hours to several weeks.

WHAT ARE THE BENEFITS OF HOSPICE CARE?

Families of individuals who received care through a hospice program are more satisfied with end-of-life care than those who did not have hospice services. Additionally, hospice recipients are more likely to have their pain controlled and are less likely to undergo tests or be given medications that they do not need, compared with people who do not use hospice care.

ADVANCE CARE PLANNING AND END-OF-LIFE DECISIONS

When a person is diagnosed with a serious illness, they should prioritize early advance care planning conversations with their family and doctors. Studies have shown that patients who participate in advance care planning are more likely to be satisfied with their care and receive care that aligns with their wishes.[1]

[1] National Institute on Aging (NIA), "What Are Palliative Care and Hospice Care?" National Institutes of Health (NIH), May 14, 2021. Available online. URL: www.nia.nih.gov/health/hospice-and-palliative-care/what-are-palliative-care-and-hospice-care. Accessed October 22, 2024.

Part 7 | Additional Help and Information

Chapter 40 | Glossary of Terms Related to the Kidney Disease and Urinary Tract Disorders

albuminuria: Presence of protein in urine.

amyloidosis: A condition in which a protein-like material builds up in one or more organs. This material cannot be broken down and interferes with the normal function of that organ.

anemia: A condition in which the body does not have enough healthy red blood cells. Red blood cells provide oxygen to body tissues.

angiotensin-converting enzyme (ACE) inhibitors: A drug that is used to lower blood pressure. An angiotensin-converting enzyme inhibitor is a type of antihypertensive agent.

angiotensin receptor blockers (ARB): Agents, such as losartan, that bind with angiotensin receptors, thus preventing access of angiotensin II to the receptor and consequently reducing the vasoconstriction produced by this agonist; used in the treatment of hypertension.

benign prostatic hyperplasia (BPH): Progressive enlargement of the prostate due to hyperplasia of both glandular and stromal components, typically beginning in the fifth decade and sometimes causing obstructive or irritative symptoms, or both; does not evolve into cancer.

This glossary contains terms excerpted from documents produced by several sources deemed reliable.

biopsy: A procedure that removes cells or tissue from your body. Pathologist looks at the cells or tissue under a microscope to check for damage or disease. The pathologist may also do other tests on it.

bladder: The balloon-shaped organ inside the pelvis that holds urine.

bladder stone: A solid mass made up of tiny crystals. One or more stones can be in the kidney or ureter at the same time.

catheter: A tubular instrument to allow passage of fluid from or into a body cavity or blood vessel. Especially a catheter designed to be passed through the urethra into the bladder to drain it of retained urine.

chronic kidney disease (CKD): Slow and progressive loss of kidney function over several years, resulting in permanent kidney failure. People with permanent kidney failure need dialysis or transplantation to replace the work of the kidneys.

clinical trial: A type of research study that uses volunteers to test new methods of screening, prevention, diagnosis, or treatment of a disease. Also called a "clinical study."

congenital: Existing at birth, referring to certain mental or physical traits, anomalies, malformations, diseases, and so on, which may be either hereditary or due to an influence occurring during gestation up to the moment of birth.

creatinine: A waste product in the blood that results from the normal breakdown of muscle. Healthy kidneys filter creatinine from the blood.

cystitis: Inflammation of the urinary bladder.

cystocele: A condition in which supportive tissues around the bladder and vaginal wall weaken and stretch, allowing the bladder and vaginal wall to fall into the vaginal canal.

diabetes: Either diabetes insipidus or diabetes mellitus, diseases having in common the symptom polyuria; when used without qualification, refers to diabetes mellitus.

dialysate: That part of a mixture that passes through a dialyzing membrane; the material that does not pass through is referred to as the retentate.

dialysis: The process of cleaning wastes from the blood artificially. This job is normally done by the kidneys. If the kidneys fail, the blood must be cleaned artificially with special equipment. The two major forms of dialysis are hemodialysis and peritoneal dialysis.

dialyzer: The apparatus for performing dialysis; a membrane used in dialysis.

edema: Swelling caused by the accumulation of fluid in cells and tissues. In kidney failure, fluid may collect in the feet, hands, abdomen, or face.

end-stage renal disease (ESRD): Total and permanent kidney failure. When the kidneys fail, the body retains fluid and harmful wastes build up. A person with ESRD needs treatment to replace the work of the failed kidneys.

***Escherichia coli* (*E. coli*)**: A species that occurs normally in the intestines of humans and other vertebrates, is widely distributed in nature, and is a frequent cause of infections of the urogenital tract and of neonatal meningitis and diarrhea in infants.

glomerulonephritis: Renal disease characterized by diffuse inflammatory changes in glomeruli that are not the acute response to infection of the kidneys.

glomerulosclerosis: Hyaline deposits or scarring within the renal glomeruli, a degenerative process occurring in association with renal arteriosclerosis or diabetes.

glomerulus: The tiny cluster of looping blood vessels in the nephron, where wastes are filtered from the blood.

hematuria: Presence of blood or red blood cells (RBCs) in the urine.

hypertension: High blood pressure (HBP), a condition that can cause kidney damage or be caused by kidney disease.

intravenous (IV): Into or within a vein. Intravenous usually refers to a way of giving a drug or other substance through a needle or tube inserted into a vein.

Kegel exercises: Alternate contraction and relaxation of perineal muscles for treatment of urinary stress incontinence.

kidneys: One of a pair of organs in the abdomen. The kidneys remove waste and extra water from the blood (as urine) and help keep chemicals (such as sodium, potassium, and calcium) balanced in the body. The kidneys also make hormones that help control blood pressure and stimulate bone marrow to make red blood cells.

nephrectomy: Surgical removal of the kidney.

nephron: One of a million tiny filtering units in each kidney. Each nephron is made up of both a glomerulus and a fluid-collecting tubule that processes extra water and wastes.

nephropathy: Any disease of the kidney.

percutaneous: Denoting the passage of substances through unbroken skin; also passage through the skin by needle puncture.

pessary: An appliance of varied form, introduced into the vagina to support the uterus or to correct any displacement.

polycystic kidney disease (PKD): A genetic disorder that causes many cysts to grow in the kidneys. PKD cysts cause high blood pressure and problems with blood vessels in the brain and heart. Cysts in the liver can also occur with PKD.

polyuria: Excessive excretion of urine resulting in profuse and frequent micturition (urination).

prostate: A gland in the male reproductive system just below the bladder. It surrounds part of the urethra, the canal that empties the bladder, and produces a fluid that forms part of semen.

prostatitis: A frequently painful condition that involves inflammation of the prostate and sometimes the areas around the prostate.

proteinuria: Large amounts of protein in the urine.

renal: Of the kidneys. A renal disease is a disease of the kidneys. Renal failure means the kidneys have stopped working properly.

renal agenesis: Absence of one or both kidneys.

renal pelvis: The area at the center of the kidney. Urine collects here and is funneled into the ureter, the tube that connects the kidney to the bladder.

stage: The extent of a cancer within the body. If the cancer has spread, the stage describes how far it has spread from the original site to other parts of the body.

staging: Performing exams and tests to learn the extent of the cancer within the body, especially whether the disease has spread from the original site to other parts of the body. It is important to know the stage of the disease in order to plan the best treatment.

transitional cell: Any cell thought to represent a phase of development from one form to another.

urea: A substance formed by the breakdown of protein in the liver. The kidneys filter urea out of the blood and into the urine. Urea can also be made in the laboratory.

ureter: The tube that conducts the urine from the renal pelvis to the bladder; it consists of an abdominal part and a pelvic part.

urethra: The canal leading from the bladder, discharging the urine externally.

urgency: A strong desire to void.

urinary tract: The body's drainage system for removing urine, which is made up of wastes and extra fluid.

urinary tract infection (UTI): Also known as "bladder infections," are most often caused by bacteria (germs) that enter the bladder, a part of the urinary tract.

urinate: To release urine from the bladder to the outside.

vascular: A general term to describe the area on the body where blood is drawn for circulation through a hemodialysis circuit. A vascular access may be an arteriovenous fistula, a graft, or a catheter.

Chapter 41 | Directory of Organizations Providing Information about Kidney Disease and Urinary Tract Disorders

GOVERNMENT ORGANIZATIONS

Centers for Disease Control and Prevention (CDC)
1600 Clifton Rd.
Atlanta, GA 30329-4027
Toll-Free: 800-CDC-INFO (800-232-4636)
Toll-Free TTY: 888-232-6348
Website: www.cdc.gov

Centers for Medicare & Medicaid Services (CMS)
7500 Security Blvd.
Baltimore, MD 21244-1850
Toll-Free: 800-MEDICARE (800-633-4227)
Phone: 410-786-3000
TTY: 410-786-0727
Toll-Free TTY: 866-226-1819
Website: www.cms.gov

Genetic and Rare Diseases Information Center (GARD)
P.O. Box 8126
Gaithersburg, MD 20898-8126
Toll-Free: 888-205-2311
Phone: 301-251-4925
Toll-Free TTY: 888-205-3223
Fax: 301-251-4911
Website: https://rarediseases.info.nih.gov

Resources in this chapter were compiled from several sources deemed reliable; all contact information was verified and updated in November 2024.

MedlinePlus
8600 Rockville Pike
Bethesda, MD 20894
Toll-Free: 888-FIND-NLM
(888-346-3656)
Phone: 301-594-5983
Website: https://medlineplus.gov

National Cancer Institute (NCI)
Toll-Free: 800-4-CANCER
(800-422-6237)
Website: www.cancer.gov
Email: NCIinfo@nih.gov

National Center for Biotechnology Information (NCBI)
8600 Rockville Pike
Bethesda, MD 20894
Website: www.ncbi.nlm.nih.gov
Email: nihms-help@ncbi.nlm.nih.gov

National Center for Complementary and Integrative Health (NCCIH)
9000 Rockville Pike
Bethesda, MD 20892
Toll-Free: 888-644-6226
Toll-Free TTY: 866-464-3615
Website: www.nccih.nih.gov
Email: info@nccih.nih.gov

National Institute of Biomedical Imaging and Bioengineering (NIBIB)
6707 Democracy Blvd., Ste. 202
Bethesda, MD 20892-5469
Phone: 301-496-8859
Website: www.nibib.nih.gov
Email: info@nibib.nih.gov

National Institute of Diabetes and Digestive and Kidney Diseases (NIDDK)
1 Information Way
Bethesda, MD 20892
Toll-Free: 800-860-8747
Toll-Free TTY: 866-569-1162
Fax: 301-634-0716
Website: www.niddk.nih.gov
Email: healthinfo@niddk.nih.gov

National Institute of Neurological Disorders and Stroke (NINDS)
P.O. Box 5801
Bethesda, MD 20824
Toll-Free: 800-352-9424
Website: www.ninds.nih.gov

National Institute on Aging (NIA)
31 Center Dr.
Bldg. 31, Rm. 5C27
Bethesda, MD 20892
Toll-Free: 800-222-2225
Website: www.nia.nih.gov
Email: niaic@nia.nih.gov

National Institutes of Health (NIH)
9000 Rockville Pike
Bethesda, MD 20892
Phone: 301-496-4000
TTY: 301-402-9612
Website: www.nih.gov

NIH News in Health
Bldg. 31, Rm. 5B52
Bethesda, MD 20892-2094
Phone: 301-451-8224
Website: https://newsinhealth.nih.gov
Email: nihnewsinhealth@od.nih.gov

Office of Disease Prevention and Health Promotion (ODPHP)
1101 Wootton Pkwy., Ste. 420
Rockville, MD 20852
Website: https://health.gov

Office on Women's Health (OWH)
1101 Wootton Pkwy.
Rockville, MD 20852
Toll-Free: 800-994-9662
Phone: 202-690-7650
Fax: 202-205-2631
Website: www.womenshealth.gov

U.S. Department of Agriculture (USDA)
1400 Independence Ave., S.W.
Washington, DC 20250
Phone: 202-720-2791
Website: www.usda.gov

U.S. Department of Veterans Affairs (VA)
Toll-Free: 800-698-2411
Website: www.va.gov

U.S. Food and Drug Administration (FDA)
10903 New Hampshire Ave.
Silver Spring, MD 20993-0002
Toll-Free: 888-INFO-FDA
(888-463-6332)
Phone: 301-796-8240
Website: www.fda.gov

PRIVATE ORGANIZATIONS

American Association of Clinical Urologists (AACU)
1061 East Main St., Ste. 300
East Dundee, IL 60118
Phone: 847-752-5355
Website: https://aacuweb.org
Email: info@aacuweb.org

American Association of Genitourinary Surgeons (AAGUS)
6545 Hwy. 54, St. 2006
Sharpsburg, GA 30277
Phone: 770-853-4001
Toll-Free Fax: 877-229-3412
Website: www.aagus.org

American Association of Kidney Patients (AAKP)
14440 Bruce B. Downs Blvd.
Tampa, FL 33613
Toll-Free: 800-749-AAKP
(800-749-2257)
Phone: 813-636-8100
Fax: 813-636-8122
Website: https://aakp.org
Email: info@aakp.org

American Board of Urology (ABU)
600 Peter Jefferson Pkwy., Ste. 150
Charlottesville, VA 22911
Phone: 434-979-0059
Website: https://abu.org
Email: info@abu.org

American Kidney Fund (AKF)
11921 Rockville Pike, Ste. 300
Rockville, MD 20852
Toll-Free: 800-638-8299
Website: www.kidneyfund.org

American Nephrology Nurses' Association (ANNA)
East Holly Ave., Box 56
Pitman, NJ 08071-0056
Toll-Free: 888-600-2662
Phone: 856-256-2320
Fax: 856-589-7463
Website: www.annanurse.org
Email: anna@annanurse.org

American Society for Histocompatibility and Immunogenetics (ASHI)
5051 Rt. 42, Unit 4, PMB 1072
Turnersville, NJ 08012
Phone: 856-335-3299
Website: www.ashi-hla.org
Email: info@ashi-hla.org

American Society of Nephrology (ASN)
1401 H St., N.W., Ste. 900
Washington, DC 20005
Phone: 202-640-4660
Fax: 202-637-9793
Website: www.asn-online.org
Email: email@asn-online.org

American Society of Pediatric Nephrology (ASPN)
6728 Old McLean Village Dr.
McLean, VA 22101
Phone: 703-884-9574
Fax: 703-556-8729
Website: https://aspneph.org
Email: info@aspneph.com

American Society of Transplant Surgeons (ASTS)
1401 South Clark St.
Ste. 1120
Arlington, VA 22202
Phone: 703-414-7870
Fax: 703-414-7874
Website: www.asts.org
Email: asts@asts.org

American Society of Transplantation (AST)
1000 Atrium Way, Ste. 400
Mt. Laurel, NJ 8054
Phone: 856-439-9986
Fax: 856-581-9604
Website: www.myast.org

American Urogynecologic Society (AUGS)
9466 Georgia Ave., PMB 2064
Silver Spring, MD 20910
Phone: 301-273-0570
Website: www.augs.org
Email: info@augs.org

Dignity Health
185 Berry St., Ste. 200
San Francisco, CA 94107
Website: www.dignityhealth.org

Endourological Society
4100 Duff Pl.
Lower Level Seaford, NY 11783
Phone: 516-520-1226
Fax: 516-520-1225
Website: www.endourology.org

International Society of Nephrology (ISN)
340 North Ave., 3rd Fl.
Cranford, NJ 07016-2496
Website: www.theisn.org
Email: info@theisn.org

International Transplant Nurses Society (ITNS)
4401 Penn Ave., Ste. 6400
Pittsburgh, PA 15301
Website: www.itns.org
Email: info@itns.org

Interstitial Cystitis Association of America, Inc. (ICA)
1660 International Dr., Ste. 600
McLean, VA 22102
Phone: 703-442-2070
Website: www.ichelp.org
Email: icamail@ichelp.org

National Association for Continence (NAFC)
2770 Arapahoe Rd., Ste. 132-1020
Lafayette, CO 80026
Toll-Free: 800-BLADDER
(800-252-3337)
Website: www.nafc.org

National Kidney Foundation (NKF)
30 East 33rd St.
New York, NY 10016
Toll-Free: 800-622-9010
Fax: 212-689-9261
Website: www.kidney.org
Email: info@kidney.org

Polycystic Kidney Disease (PKD) Foundation
1001 E. 101st Terr.
Ste. 220
Kansas City, MO 64131
Toll-Free: 800-PKD-CURE
(800-753-2873)
Phone: 816-931-2600
Website: https://pkdcure.org
Email: pkdcure@pkdcure.org

Transplant Recipient International Organization (TRIO)
17560 Buckingham Garden Dr.
Lithia, FL 33547
Phone: 813-800-TRIO
(813-800-8746)
Website: www.trioweb.org
Email: info@trioweb.org

United Network for Organ Sharing (UNOS)
700 N. 4th St.
Richmond, VA 23219
Toll-Free: 800-292-9548
Phone: 804-782-4800
Website: https://unos.org

INDEX

INDEX

Page numbers followed by "n" refer to citation information; by "t" indicate tables; and by "f" indicate figures.

A

B

C

D

E

F

G

H

I

K

N

R

U

V

W

X

Z